Integrating Primary Health Care

Care

Leading, Managing, Facilitating

Paul Thomas

Professor of Primary Care Research, Education and Development
Centre for the Study of Policy & Practice in Health and Social Care
Thames Valley University

Forewords by

Mayur Lakhani

Kurt C Stange

and

David Colin-Thomé

Radcliffe Publishing
Oxford • Seattle

Radcliffe Publishing Ltd
18 Marcham Road
Abingdon
Oxon OX14 1AA
United Kingdom

www.radcliffe-oxford.com
Electronic catalogue and worldwide online ordering facility.

British Library Cataloguing in Publication Data

A catalogue record for this book is available from the British Library.

ISBN-10 1 85775 662 2
ISBN-13 978 1 85775 662 3

Typeset by Anne Joshua & Associates, Oxford
Printed and bound by TJ International Ltd, Padstow, Cornwall

I dedicate this work to the memory of Mario Kawayawaya. A one-time expert elephant poacher in Southern Zambia, he became a facilitator to preserve the African elephant. We debated facilitation methods in a series of conversations in 1994. I learnt that what he had to do to help local people, police and poachers to see each other's points of view and work together was very similar to what I had to do to develop primary care in England. In May 2004 he was paddling his canoe along the Kafue river when his spleen ruptured from malaria.

He died. Zambia lost a fine facilitator.

Contents

Foreword

This is a sophisticated book that addresses the important issue of integration in health care. It is particularly timely coming as it does in the context of the new health and social care White Paper for England, *Our Health, Our Care, Our Say*, which signals a decisive shift away from hospitals to primary care. But this begs a question: how can primary care be developed to respond to all that is being asked of it? This is a critical question for the health community. One thing is for sure – it will not happen by chance! The improvements that patients need require the extraordinary potential of primary care to be realised. This will require a major cultural change and support for the primary care community to deliver. The ingredients necessary for this exciting transformation are described in this book.

Paul Thomas's book contains information about leadership, transformation, facilitation, support, systems development, learning organisation and much more. I am in no doubt that effective integrated primary health care is the answer to many of the problems facing health care worldwide. But a lot of lip service is paid to integration in health care. What is integration? What does it look like? How do you know you have got it? It is a word like 'teams' that is bandied around with superficial discussion. This book changes this: it offers a compre-hensive analysis of the theory and practice of integration in health care. The author argues powerfully for the need for approaches that include both vertical and horizontal integration.

This is one of the most powerful books I have read. It offers well reasoned and researched ideas for improving primary care. Above all what comes through is the author's sense of passion about the subject and issues, and a sense of credibility from having being in the front line and undertaken practical work in the area.

This is a serious book tackling a serious subject. In my view it is required reading for anyone interested in or involved in primary care development.

As a practising GP, I know the problems that my patients face. As Chairman of the RCGP, and with experience of being a leader in primary care organisations, I am well aware of the problems facing general practice. Through extensive practice visits I have come to the conclusion that general practice needs to become more strategic. If we are to fulfil our 'extraordinary potential' that Paul Thomas writes about, then general practice-based primary care has to move 'up a gear'. Key to this is to develop strategic learning organisations in primary care.

The Royal College of GPs was established in 1952 and is charged with promoting the highest possible standards of general medical practice. I am particularly pleased to welcome this book as the author is also the chairman of one of the college's faculties.

The college is in the business of driving up standards, and core to this is the development of optimal team working and skill mix. GPs are the backbone of the NHS. Most GPs I meet wish they had longer consultation times, responsive access systems and could promote greater patient enablement. To achieve this we have to think creatively about the organisation of primary health and social care and Paul's book helps us do just that.

Dr Mayur Lakhani FRCGP
Chairman
Royal College of General Practitioners
January 2006

Foreword

This is an important book. It is important because of the *ideas* it contains, the *time* in which it appears, and the *grounding* of the ideas in rich practical lived experience and in theory. Readers of this book will be well-armed to make sense of challenging paradoxes and to work to improve health care and health. Although focused on primary care, health care systems and community, this work is relevant to anyone trying to bring together individuals and groups to become learning organizations moving toward a larger end.

The *ideas* in this book show very practical and realistic ways to bring together individuals and groups to become whole systems – learning organizations moving toward an emerging shared goal. Uniquely, the book is about how multiple systems can interact and evolve together toward a better whole. The first and third parts of the book help us to understand the potential of integrated primary health care and to think differently about how it really works. The second and fourth sections show us how to act on that understanding to effect change. Throughout, the author stimulates us to deepen our learning and actions by applying the ideas to our own experience.

The *time* is right for these ideas. We are experiencing a crisis of fragmentation in health care. Although we vaguely recognize the complexity of health care, as individuals and as organizations we act as if working harder on the parts is somehow going to improve the whole. It has not and will not. The phenomena of health and health care are too complex to be understood and improved solely by linear thinking. In this book, Professor Thomas shows us how we are all leaders of change, and how by working on our parts, while appreciating and developing their essential interconnectedness, we can improve the whole.

This book is *grounded* in the author's deep experience as a facilitator of whole systems change. He presents an explanatory theory that is breathtakingly integrative yet immensely practical. It is all the more powerful because it is deeply grounded in personal experience. Practice without theory is unable to move beyond isolated experiences to draw the overarching lessons. Theory without practice blinds us to the ways of knowing that don't fit our paradigm. Professor Thomas's work to discover theories that fit his radical experience of systems change gives us new ways of thinking and acting that bring together both practical experience and overarching lessons.

Join me in using this book as a springboard to 'travel hopefully' together toward integrated, equitable and effective health care.

Kurt C Stange MD, PhD
Editor, *Annals of Family Medicine*
Gertrude Donnelly Hess, MD Professor of Oncology Research
Professor of Family Medicine, Epidemiology & Biostatistics, Sociology and Oncology
Case Western Reserve University
Cleveland, Ohio, USA
January 2006

Foreword

This is a 'must-read' book if you are in any way involved in the development of primary care. It has something for everyone – both practical and theoretical – with an appropriate focus on an underpinning philosophy. I particularly enjoyed reading Part III, but would recommend that, first, read the whole and then focus on relevant parts for future use. The book is very well cross-referenced.

Integrating Primary Health Care is extremely relevant to the present as well as the future, given the centrality of primary care and health care in many countries. All primary care organisations (including general practice) have populations for which they are responsible. They should all be viewed as resources for their communities: delivering high-quality bioclinical care while addressing broader community needs.

The English White Paper links primary health care, public health and social care. This book references and explores the Alma Ata declaration and I believe that we in primary care, in particular now in England, have a unique opportunity to deliver on this declaration by linking treatment, care, the enablement of individuals and addressing the social determinants of health.

I particularly like the author's view that if we are to deliver on such an agenda we need to embrace managerial approaches that traditionally are perceived as inimical. For instance, Paul Thomas cites the need for both linear management and system reform. I suggest that other related areas which are seen as in conflict similarly need to be embraced: transactional and transformational leadership and, at a practical level, that urgent and planned care are inextricably linked. In a similar vein, I do not see localities as the only way forward for practice-based commissioning. We need a more 'organic' approach, in which activity can be based at either practice or locality level depending on what is best for patients. As is much quoted: form should follow function.

I write in a personal capacity as a general practitioner, a Department of Health worker (for England), and as a colleague and a friend of the author. I have been fortunate to be a small part of Paul's journey of discovery. This excellent book, which I thoroughly recommend, is a fitting product of that journey. Knowing the author there will be more.

David Colin-Thomé
National Clinical Director for Primary Care, Department of Health (England)
General Practitioner, Castlefields, Runcorn, Cheshire
January 2006

Preface

My childhood in South Wales taught me that communities and individuals grow together. Economic hardship and high levels of disease can also be associated with strong community identity, friendship and song. The social role of the general practitioner (GP) was also obvious to me. My father, a GP who worked alone, would watch from our house the crowds leaving the football ground, observing his patients and anticipating who would knock on his door later in the week. Once when there was a smallpox scare but no vaccine he ordered his own supply from Cardiff and travelled there to buy it, rather than wait for the local Executive Council to provide it. He and my mother immunised queues of people in the street for no charge. I was eight when he died, and, two years later, my mother took me to England with my older brother and four younger sisters. The seeds that led to this book were planted at an early age.

At school I became enthralled by relativity theory and puzzled how it was that things can, at the same time, have tangible, objective form and also be made up of dynamic energy. An interest in what lies beyond the immediately visible has been with me ever since. As a GP myself I often ask patients what they make of their symptoms and what is the best thing to do. I often receive wise and thoughtful answers that make me realise the power of 'common sense' – a sophisticated process of pattern recognition. I also witness the extraordinary ability of the human mind to overcome all kinds of adversity, and the need we all have for trusted relationships to define ourselves.

But I was trained to think in straight lines about compartmentalised problems: discrete diseases are caused by malicious agents that laboratory science can defeat. This training offered me little insight into the interplay of forces that improve health in most situations. My training also expects me to listen and reflect, solely to get to a correct diagnosis or to ensure patient compliance. I also recognise that listening and reflection can reveal hidden worlds of meaning that are barred from me if I assume in advance what I am going to find.

It was as primary care facilitator in Liverpool that I recognised that hidden worlds of meaning powerfully affect what happens in all human situations. When working across boundaries it became clear to me that different people use words to mean different things, and what they really mean is often hidden even from themselves. I often found it easier to make progress by putting aside words and theories, and getting people to play together and create shared 'win–win' projects. I slowly found resonance with the ideas about change I was developing – in complexity and systems theories, organisational learning and narrative. Slowly I began to see coherent patterns within dynamic interactivity, like a beautiful form of music whose beat and harmonies are new, but also very familiar and human.

I came to see that quality comes from reflecting one thing against another in search of coherence – reflecting internal against external realities, subjective against objective interpretations and theory against practice. This helps to avoid assumptions. It promotes active listening and ongoing learning. It helps to recognise that the more you know the more you know you don't know. It reminds us that the path ahead is uncertain and we have to work hard to make it meaningful.

Finding a meaningful path through uncertainty is what leaders do in complex situations. Will Miller gave me an image to illuminate this. It is the walk of the Lenape Native American Indian. Balanced and relaxed on one foot, alert and listening with all the senses, progress is achieved by cautiously testing the safety of the ground ahead with the toes of the other foot. When it seems safe, a step is softly taken, slowly transferring weight onto the front foot. The front foot is now the one balanced in safety. Again listening with all the senses, and communicating with groups of colleagues about the overall direction, each prepares their next step in their own individual but connected way.

I wish you an enjoyable walk.

Paul Thomas
January 2006

About the author

Dr Paul Thomas graduated at Bristol University in 1979. In 1986 he became a general practitioner (GP) at Princes Park Health Centre, Toxteth, Liverpool, which is famous for its community involvement and patient participation. In 1989 he became a primary care facilitator for Liverpool Family Health Services Authority and translated the holistic ideals of his practice – of multidisciplinary learning – into multiple models throughout the city, working closely with the Liverpool Healthy City 2000 project.

In 1996 Paul was appointed as senior lecturer at Imperial College in London, from where he set up the West London (Primary Care) Research Network and chaired the Advisory Group for the National Primary Care Facilitation Project. In 2003 he was awarded a MD for his thesis: whole-system learning and change – the role of primary care research networks. In 2004 Paul was awarded Fellowship of the Royal College of General Practitioners (RCGP). In his role as Chair of the North and West London Faculty of the RCGP and as a professor at Thames Valley University he continues to develop leadership programmes for integrated primary care.

Acknowledgements

I learnt how to do most of this in Liverpool. I owe thanks to the thousands of people in the hundreds of teams with whom I worked in those 10 years. In particular, I remember with affection the contributions to my learning of members of the Primary Care Facilitation Project, Medical Audit Advisory Group and the practice teams with whom we worked. I remember teams from Princes Park Health Centre, Liverpool Health Authority and the Family Health Services Authority, the Liverpool Occupational Health Project, local multidisciplinary facilitation teams, the Teambuilding Workshop Local Organising Group, the Healthy City 2000 Project, the Heart Disease Strategy Group, the Liverpool City of Learning, Age Concern, the community health council, Open Eye Film and Video Gallery, the John Moores Centre for Health Studies, and Liverpool University departments of General Practice, Public Health and Nursing. I enjoyed finding like-minded people through the Association of General Practice in Urban Deprived Areas, the Health Education Authority, the Oxford Primary Care Facilitation Project, the King's Fund and the Royal College of General Practitioners (RCGP) Health Inequalities Standing Group.

I especially remember the fun I had trying to work it all out with Janet Hayes, Cathy Hogan, Annette James, Conan Leavey, Helena Lunt, Len Ratoff, Gill Ridpath, Rose Sands, Janet Snodden, Claire Vile, and Sheila and her friends.

I learnt how to express the ideas mainly in London. In addition to the above, I have been fortunate to have had my thinking challenged and stretched by Louise Acheson, Jen Anderson, Franklin Apfel, Richard Ashcroft, Ricky Banarsee, Fritjof Capra, Peter Cawley, Siobhan Clarke, David Colin-Thomé, Ben Crabtree, Vicky Doyle, Chris Dowrick, Charles Easmon, Ewan Ferlie, Rosemary Field, Madeleine Gantley, Steve Gillam, Pat Gordon, Jonathan Graffy, Susanna Graham-Jones, Frances Griffiths, Iona Heath, John Horder, Ray Ison, Joe Kai, Maurice Keane, John Launer, Lou Lukas, John MacDonald, Lynne Madden, Janette McCulloch, Will Miller, Sue Morrison, David Nabarro, Aislinn O'Dwyer, Mike Parker, Diane Plamping, Julian Pratt, Paul Quin, Peter Sainsbury, Patricia Shaw, Ralph Stacey, Susan Weil, Alison While and my many new friends at Thames Valley University (London, UK). Many also helped with the presentation of ideas.

I owe special thanks to Peter Kinch, Gillian Nineham and Kurt Stange, who were with me at every stage of writing this book. I am not sure I would have got there without you.

I want to thank my mother, Wendy, for having such courage and being such an inspiration to me, and thanks to my brother Michael and sisters Manda, Gaynor, Anne and Nonita.

I want to thank my father Ronald – I know you would have been proud of all of us.

I also want to thank my beautiful wife Eunice, and our children David and Peter.

How to use this book

There are many possible paths through this book, and simply reading it from beginning to end may not be the most helpful one. The book is a map of the practical and theoretical things that I have found important to understand how to integrate different efforts for health. Key to grounding this knowledge in (your) everyday practice is moving between theory and experience. The book is intended to facilitate this movement.

In addition to the Contents, the following are intended to help you to find your best path.

- A summary at the beginning of each chapter – you may like to read these first to get a feel of the whole book.
- Images and models – in Chapter 2 and in chapters 4–8 I propose images and models that may help you to catch the ideas better than the text. You may wish to view these first.
- Examples, practical things to do and exercises – these are included throughout Part II and may help you to find a focus for your reading.
- Connecting theory and practice – Parts I and III of the book are concerned largely with theory; parts II and IV are concerned with practice. I cross-refer so that you can move between them.
- Pause – these prompt you to pause and reflect on how you make sense of something. Doing this gives you a chance to disagree with my interpretation, and also to skip whole sections that are not presently a priority for you to explore.

The four parts of the book have different purposes:

- Part I explains why integrated primary health care is important.
- Part II helps you to develop leadership skills.
- Part III explores theories of integration.
- Part IV describes useful techniques.

Read Part I if you want to know why this is important It maps the territory, discusses the meaning of leadership and explores the potential of contemporary health care. In Chapter 1, I begin a discussion of power, identity and culture, which is continued in Part III.

Read Part II if you want to develop your leadership skills. In each chapter I pose three evolving scenarios: the development of a general practice; the development of a community hospital; and locality development. You are invited to choose the closest to your real-life experience. The scenarios reflect three different kinds of organisation:

- A small enterprise that comprises a multidisciplinary team with shared vision and plans.
- A large institution that houses multiple semi-independent programmes of work.
- A network where members dip in and out of many activities depending on their interest at the time (the idea of a network as an organisation may be unfamiliar, but bear with me).

At the start of each chapter I pose a new twist to the stories and invite you to describe how you would deal with this. At the end of the chapter I ask whether the chapter has helped you to think differently about your plan, and what you have learnt.

Read Part III if you want theory about integration. People are complex, semi-independent but also inter-dependent. Facilitating integration, like 'herding cats', is not straightforward. I first relate integrated primary health care to the idea of 'comprehensive primary health care' as envisaged by the World Health Organization (WHO), and also to generalist practice (medical and otherwise). I then highlight changes needed in our understanding of science, health and change, to better understand how to think about integrated health care. I argue in each situation how linear thinking and systems thinking offer different insights into the whole.

Read Part IV if you want to learn techniques that help to see parts and wholes at the same time. They can be used in different situations to help people to 'see' how their work is relevant to bigger, evolving stories.

What I mean by . . .

This list includes abbreviations and the meaning I have attached to certain terms.

General practice/practitioners (GP) – this term, from the UK, is equivalent to 'family physicians' in the USA. These are medically trained practitioners who mainly operate outside of hospitals, are often the first port of call for people with health problems, usually work in multidisciplinary teams, and are responsible for orchestrating a diversity of support for health needs.

Integrated primary health care – this term comes from contemporary health care. It remains to be seen if this will be more like comprehensive or selective primary health care.

Leader – an individual who helps people (perhaps a named constituency) to move forwards.

Leaders, managers and facilitators – these roles have traditionally been distinguished in a linear way: a *leader* shows the way; a *manager* makes things happen; a *facilitator* eases the process. But in complex situations these distinctions are blurred. Leaders cannot avoid considering how ideas can be applied practically, managers cannot avoid inspiring and wisely directing people, and facilitators need vision and political sensitivity to know how far to allow people to deviate from a pre-ordained path.

Leadership for integrated primary health care – also includes the leadership teams, networks and an array of resources and agreements needed to move forwards a whole story.

Organisation – in its broadest sense this means any way of organising people that produces a collective identity. In particular, I use the terms *institution, small/medium-sized enterprise (SME)* and *network* to show how different organisational types have different strengths and weaknesses.

Primary care – this means more than general practice and less than primary health care.

Primary care organisation (PCO) – this includes any organisation that considers itself to be part of primary care, for example general practices, dentists, pharmacists. PCOs are statutory network organisations in the UK, termed **primary care trusts (PCTs)** in England. They have a role to integrate a diversity of services.

Primary health care (PHC) – this is the term used by the World Health Organization (WHO) at the 1978 conference of Alma Ata. It means that all aspects of society and all citizens have a responsibility for health. Medical practitioners contribute an important part, but it is only a part. *Comprehensive PHC* includes horizontal and vertical integration of effort. *Selective PHC* means vertical integration of effort only.

Theories in use: mental models, mindsets, personal constructs, hidden motivations – these terms have different origins, but all describe the subconscious ideas that guide the ways in which people think and act. These are often more powerful that what people actually say.

Part I

Why integrated primary health care is important

Part I explains why integrated primary health care is important, and offers some challenges to achieving it.

Chapter 1 provides an overview of the ideas being put forward. Leadership is described as making sense within complexity. A discussion of power, identity and culture is also begun, and is continued in Part III.

Chapter 2 puts some flesh on the bones of this image of leadership, pointing towards Part II, in which leadership skills are developed, and Part IV, in which useful techniques are described.

Chapter 3 signposts ways to achieve long-term integration of primary health care, in particular by applying the principles of a learning organisation to health care localities.

Chapter 1

Mapping the territory

Summary

This book is concerned with ongoing and co-ordinated behaviour change – how do you energise people from different organisations and backgrounds to ask important questions, reflect on the implications of the knowledge they generate and change things in concert.

The ideas are particularly useful for leaders, managers, facilitators and others who help people to move forwards in complex situations. In these situations many things are changing constantly, and predictions are far less certain than in simple situations.

I use the term 'leader' to mean an individual who helps people (perhaps a named constituency) to move forwards. By contrast, 'leadership for integrated primary health care' also includes the leadership teams, networks and array of resources and agreements needed to move forwards a whole 'story'.

Leaders help people to make sense of their work within bigger pictures. Leadership makes learning in one part of the system relevant to other parts through 'whole-system conversations'. I paint a picture of the world through a constructivist lens – everything is undergoing ongoing adaptation to everything else, and what you see largely depends on the way you look. This notion recognises the limitation of words to represent experience. It recognises that mental models which determine behaviour are often hidden from view even from the people involved.

Leadership helps people to think for themselves and to learn from others. It helps them to apply knowledge from elsewhere wisely and to generate their own insights. It helps them to modify their plans to fit better with those of others. It is concerned with long-term as well as short-term success; with discrete focused activity as well as whole-system transformation.

Leadership is first concerned with using existing structures better. Wholly new structures may not be needed. It helps people to use time differently to save time overall, and also to produce better outcomes. It helps people to develop thoughtful, strategic plans that can accommodate multiple agendas, rather than adopting an overly reactive and rushed approach.

I use the term 'integrated' to mean that different efforts for health are constantly made relevant to each other. I do not mean that everything is 'hard-wired' into everything else. Leadership creates pathways to 'learning spaces' where people with different insights and traditions come together to find common purpose and develop collaborative projects.

Vertical integration includes care pathways for named diseases. Horizontal integration includes multi-disciplinary team-working across organisational boundaries. The concepts of whole systems, organisational learning and shared leadership help us to think about achieving vertical and horizontal integration at the same time.

Whole-system change can be uncomfortable for those who think mainly in linear ways because it achieves things that their dominant mental model considers impossible. The skills of leadership are similar to the skills of systems practice and mature citizenship. All recognise that parts and wholes must co-evolve and remain relevant to each other, and that things always work out differently to what was expected. Leaders are less certain about final destinations and divert more energy to helping people to travel hopefully.

Is this book for you?

Pause

Why are you interested in leadership for integrated primary health care?

This book will help you to be a systems practitioner, able to make different efforts for health come together as integrated wholes. You do this by connecting learning spaces in which multi-disciplinary groups share their insights and align their agendas. This is a process that builds 'learning communities' and coherent whole systems of care.

Parts II and IV of the book will be most useful to practitioners and managers who facilitate integration of diverse efforts for health – in these I suggest that whole-system learning and change can be viewed as play, and leaders as story-weavers.

Teachers and theorists about complexity and organisational learning may find the theory of Parts I and III helpful – in these I describe a clash of ideologies between linear and systems thinking, which can be resolved by moving between the two.

This book is targeted at those who lead change in health care institutions such as primary care organisations (PCOs) (a statutory UK organisation, termed primary care trusts (PCTs) in England), in smaller PCOs, such as general practices, and in networks. In particular, the book explores leadership in complex situations where many things are changing at the same time. In contrast to simple situations, what happens as a result of an action in complex situations is often unpredictable.

In complex situations leaders are first concerned with bringing into view existing structures and resources, inviting participants to use these better. Later they use the energy from good group process to create new connections between existing structures (and sometimes wholly new entities). Leaders help people to use time differently in order to save time and also to produce better outcomes. They help people to develop thoughtful strategic plans which can accommodate multiple agendas, rather than adopting an overly reactive and rushed approach.

I include in the term 'leader' those people who are effective at helping certain constituencies to integrate primary health care. I consider 'leadership' to include these individuals, and the leadership teams, networks and array of resources and agreements that are together needed to move forwards a whole story in a healthy way.

The roles of leader, manager and facilitator have traditionally been separated in a linear way – a leader to show the way, a manager to make things happen, a facilitator to ease the process. But in complex situations these distinctions obstruct understanding. 'Leaders' cannot avoid considering how ideas can be practically applied. 'Managers' cannot avoid inspiring and wisely directing people. 'Facilitators' need vision and political sensitivity to know how far to allow people to deviate from a pre-ordained path.

The language of leadership, management and facilitation originally arose from a time when it was thought that the world could be explained in terms of Newtonian 'particle' physics – discrete particles are ordered in an enduring and predictable way. Consequently it was natural to think in a 'linear' way – a knight in shining armour would lead change in a direct way and make simple distinctions between right and wrong, confident that other things would stay the same. However, we now recognise that this 'laboratory' understanding of knowledge does not apply when many factors interact. Instead we must consider more interactive theories of knowledge and change: for example, relativity physics and complexity theory, which recognise that things are more interconnected, co-adapting and uncertain than they appear at first sight. Everything is changing internally, and everything is adapting to changes in everything else.

The newness of ideas about complex adaptation means that the theoretical base of leadership within it is uncertain. I use theories and models from various places throughout the book but it is also my intention to contribute to theory-building. This is most evident in Part III. I use the term 'primary health care' to mean the vision of Alma Ata that all citizens and all aspects of society have a role in improving health (Chapter 9). The term 'primary care' emerged in the 1980s to mean more than general practice and less than primary health care. I use the term 'integrated' to mean that different efforts for health are constantly made relevant to each other. I do not mean that everything should be 'hard-wired' together, or that a final complete state of integration is possible or desirable. Instead, leaders are concerned with creating pathways between different efforts for health and care. These lead to 'learning spaces' where people with different insights and traditions come together to find common purpose. Stability comes not from a giant template for change, but from ongoing cycles of cross-organisational reflection and action. These make it easier for individuals and groups to adapt to the changes in others in the most useful ways. The constraints on change come less from control from above, and more from the capacity of people to make new alliances.

Vertical integration includes care pathways. Horizontal integration includes multi-disciplinary team-working across organisational boundaries. Both are needed. I emphasise general practice partly because most of my work has involved general practitioners (GPs) (and I am one). However, I also think that generalist roles (not just medical) are an essential part of integrated primary health care and this potential has yet to be fully realised. I devote Chapter 10 to the origins and potential of general medical practice.

I am not covering the mechanisms that organisations create to control others, because these are amply covered elsewhere. I am also not covering psychometric tools such as Belbin team roles, Honey and Mumford (Kolb) learning styles and Myers Briggs personality types. I concentrate on co-ordinated reflection and action – how to energise teams from different organisations and backgrounds to learn and change things in concert. I describe successful models, especially in Part II, as examples of what happens when people of different backgrounds configure services that make sense to them and their own local context. In particular I emphasise different ways to connect enquiry and action. These are basic elements of (Kolb's) learning cycle.[1] Individuals, organisations and systems learn by asking good questions, generating appropriate data, and then reflecting on the implications of what they find to next steps. This idea shows how to connect experience and ideas for an individual through reflective practice,[2] and action learning,[3] and for groups and organisations through participatory action research[4] and 'R&D systems'.[5] It leads to Senge's idea of a learning organisation,[6] Wenger's idea of a learning community[7] and Cooperider's idea of appreciative inquiry.[8,9] It leads to the three quite different types of learning as described by Argyris and Schon.[10]

I suggest ways to think about leaders and leadership, and offer practical things to do. Mostly these do not require extra resources. However, they do require you to play – to engage with others, listen carefully to them, see things from their point of view, and to reflect their ideas against yours to find new imaginative ways forward. Part IV describes techniques to do this. It entails living with uncertainty because you know that things will always work out differently from the original intention. Success needs people to try out new ways of doing things and review the lessons learnt from many innovations as a whole, each player modifying their steps to fit better with others. Part II describes skills and models to lead this.

I will have achieved my aim if this book helps you to keep your eyes fixed on effective ways forward in the middle of multiple forces that threaten to knock you off balance, and attractive diversions that will lead into blind alleys. The book will not tell you exactly what to do, but it will help you to shape a winning approach.

Why the book has a non-linear structure

In the 'How to use the book' section I describe features to help you navigate the text in the way that best suits you. This is needed because I conclude that neither theory nor practice can understand leadership within complexity – ongoing movement between both is needed. I wish to facilitate your movement, and work from your own experience.

I paint a picture of the world through a constructivist lens (Chapter 11), everything is undergoing ongoing adaptation to everything else, and what you see largely depends on the way you look. The relativistic and dynamic theories to make sense of this are explored in Part III. I conclude the following, which guide the structure of the book.

- Words, theories and objective facts mark something meaningful, but this meaning is much more bound to the context of its origin than the words/theories/facts can portray (Chapter 11). Theory is necessarily a thin extraction from more interconnected truths. It is therefore insufficient to start with one theoretical position and simply move from there to its practical implications.

- Everyone's experience is unique, and bound into their own complex and evolving story (Chapter 12). Often, the most important motivating factors for behaviour are hidden and 'undiscussable' (Chapter 13). Furthermore, both experience and common sense are not discrete things but a complex coming together of many different senses (in Chapter 11 I use the image of a gardener who uses various senses to experience a garden). It is therefore insufficient to start with one experience and simply move to its theoretical implications.
- There is a reliable starting point – each person wishes to describe his or her life stories as a coherent narrative (Chapter 12). This suggests that you, the reader, should bring your own stories to the book, and I should bring mine. To assist this I ask you to pause at various places to consider your own interests and understandings. I signpost different parts of the book to help you to move about in ways that make sense to you.

The emphasis of this book is on the dynamic processes of whole-system learning and change, and leadership that enables this. But, stable organisations are also important to support and protect network activity, in the same way a spider needs stable structures on which to attach its web.

An image that reveals this hard/dynamic tension is an iceberg (thanks to Louis Acheson for this image). Reality, as we perceive it, really does have hard shape (as does an iceberg). The ice is tangible, amenable to objective scientific testing and has predictable behaviour. However, this hard reality is not the starting point. It is an endpoint (at least for now). The 'starting point' (and the term has doubtful meaning) may be the complex interactions between ice, water, temperature and salts at the edges of the iceberg. And every small part of its edges has a different shape from all the other parts, its own micro-climate and influential local factors. The edges are constantly changing shape, which, in time, change the shape of the whole iceberg. Leadership for integrated primary health care works at the edges, mindful of the whole. So I am inviting you to play. You bring your experiences and ideas, and I bring mine. We are both trying to make sense of our very different experiences. Let us see what agreements, disagreements and new insights we can find by travelling together for a while.

What is leadership for integrated primary health care?

> **Pause**
>
> *What do you mean by leadership for integrated primary health care?*

Leadership for integrated health care is, naturally enough, concerned with processes of integration – it helps people to value different ideas about the way things should be, and help them to find win–win ways forward. The leadership image is less that of a pioneer cowboy carving a lonely path through uncharted territory, and more that of a facilitator in the tower of Babel, holding the space for different people to listen to each other, and, from this listening, to learn, find common purpose and take tentative steps in synchrony. There is still a need for heroic individuals who lead 'followers' in new directions, but such leaders are equally concerned with empowering those followers to think for themselves and reflect on the impact of their actions on the whole system.

This form of leadership helps people to learn from others and to develop systems with multiple purposes, to avoid duplicating effort and re-inventing wheels. It helps people to think for themselves as skilled listeners and reflective practitioners, so they can wisely apply knowledge from other places to the specific context. It is concerned with sustainable evolution of individual organisations and systems, and policy for both the long and the short term. For the long term it builds an infrastructure of facilitation and communication – this helps people to constantly redefine their trajectory in the context of a longer-term story. For the short term it helps them to carry out innovative projects that will test the next steps. It is fundamentally concerned with equity – fairness. This is not to imagine that everyone is the same, but that everyone can and should learn from others, and each person is to be respected for who they are as a whole human being.

Integrated primary health care requires widespread recognition that discrete actions can have unpredictable effects on whole systems of care (remember the chaos theory butterfly that flapped its wings and caused a hurricane the other side of the world). Immediate effects, which we prize so highly, may not be the most important or sustainable effects – they may even be harmful in the long run. Change requires new relationships between those who are connected in a system of care. Without this, things will go back to where they were before.

An individual leader relates to a 'constituency' – people who recognise the person as a leader to help them move forwards, making sense of their work to bigger pictures. Sometimes the constituency comprises a discrete group or discipline, sometimes it is a geographic area and sometimes it is those who share an idea. Leaders keep in touch with their constituencies.

Sometimes leaders have formal roles, such as chief executives. But there are leaders everywhere, going by much more modest titles, and doing things that at first sight might seem unimportant. Most do not even recognise themselves to be leaders. Often, they are the quiet people who just seem to be wise, or the glue that keeps things together. They are concerned with long-term vision as well as with immediate practical details. They are patient with those who struggle to make things work, and impatient with those who do not try.

Leadership, from both individuals and teams, motivates others to think and act creatively at the cusp between the known and unknown. It helps to make it safe for people to take calculated risks, and to explore ways to advance their organisations and local services at the same time as developing themselves.

Leadership is concerned that whole systems learn and change. At any moment they may be focused on a discrete project, but they are also mindful of the other changes that need to happen, and how the stakeholders – those who have a stake in a project – can 'own' the changes.

Leadership uses techniques that help people to see bigger pictures and to make learning in one part of the system relevant to other parts. Leadership listens more than tells, reaches out more than retracts and is calm when others panic. In the terms of this book you are a leader, whether you like it or not, if this is what you do.

Leadership works with multiple motivations and multiple stories

People are the way they are for many reasons. Nature, nurture and context all influence the ways in which people think and behave. There are many motivations for learning and change, and specific motivators cannot reliably be predicted at a distance. Paying people money is not enough for the scale of engagement required by integrated primary health care (but it is an important part). Leaders work with multiple motivations to create a better future. They encourage people to find things in others to like, and then build shared projects from these things. They put people into situations where they are likely to succeed. They play to people's strengths – someone who is strong and quick to anger may not be the one to facilitate delicate negotiations, but may be ideal when it comes to a fight!

People are motivated when they can travel from wherever they are to a destination that they choose and like. Some of the motivation comes from the very process of reflecting and purposefully making this choice. Some of the motivation comes from the enjoyment of travel and the relief of arriving. It is therefore often a winning strategy to help people to describe their future vision and develop exploratory projects that help them move towards this. It also helps to provide a series of opportunities for travellers to meet again and tell their stories, reflecting on what they have learnt, and plan changes accordingly.

This process of ongoing learning and review among a group of travellers is a feature of a 'learning organisation'. It entails using time differently – less reacting to events and more team-planning, systems thinking and multi-disciplinary review of progress.

You probably already know these things. But the temptation to react to never-ending crises and to fill time with noise may prevent doing them systematically. Some people are tempted to devise grand plans to change everything in one go. At the other extreme some wish to go only one step at a time, hoping that good process will produce sustainable structures. Both of these approaches are less effective than an approach that constantly moves between long-term vision, short-term success and practical infrastructure to support both. This entails moving forward, then pausing to listen, reflect and learn, with relevant teams, about long-term and short-term infrastructure – before moving forwards again. This book shows how to develop this reflective, optimistic and incremental approach to integrated primary health care.

What leadership theorists say

Pause

What theories of leadership do you use – and why?

Children used to be told when crossing the road: 'Look right, look left, and look right again; if all is clear walk smartly to the other side'. When too many children were run over, the advice changed to 'Stop, look and listen – keep looking, keep looking – to the right and the left, forward and backwards . . . and when you get to the other side don't be too sure that it is safe'.

Sadler describes different definitions of leadership:

> . . . a process of persuasion, a set of activities, reciprocal processes of mobilisation, influencing the objectives and culture of organisations, influence processes, and 'the ability to get men to do what they don't want to do and like it.'[11]

Sadler refers to Bennis' and Nanus' three features of leadership:

1 Facing the challenge of overcoming resistance to change.
2 Brokering the needs of constituencies both within and without the organisation.
3 Being responsible for the set of ethics or norms that govern the behaviour of people in an organisation.[11]

But these features describe leadership from the perspective of one organisation in competition with others. In the context of 'leadership for integration', Bennis' and Nanus' features need to be rephrased from the perspective of many. Leadership must give rise to win–win agreements if the various players are to continue to play. A rephrasing might be:

1 Facing the challenge to get different constituencies to recognise their shared concerns, and address them in a collaborative way.
2 Brokering coalitions of interest between different constituencies to undertake shared projects that move towards their shared vision.
3 Clarifying what are the ground rules of engagement and shared vision for ethical behaviour.

This form of leadership has been called 'brokerage' in higher education:

> . . . a means of promoting and facilitating complex learning and change . . . Organizational brokering is an intentional act . . . to work in collaborative and creating ways with people, ideas, knowledge and resources to develop something new or change something.[12]

This suggests that leadership for integration facilitates shared meaning.

Weick considers a leader to be a 'sense-maker'[13] – helping people to make sense of their situations. Sense-makers trust that people will change when it is meaningful to them. They consider that people do not so much need to be told what to do, as empowered to do it.

He describes situations where named threats can quickly escalate out of control, and situations where there is a more complex array of threats and opportunities. To illustrate situations where getting things wrong can result in disaster, Weick examines the behaviour of the teams that help aircraft on and off aircraft carriers. He concludes that the characteristics of aircraft carriers which have fewer than their fair share of accidents is 'mindfulness'.[14] Mindfulness includes:

- preoccupation with failure
- reluctance to simplify interpretations
- sensitivity to operations
- commitment to resilience
- deference to expertise.

Conversely, when immediate disaster is not a concern, and instead a complex interplay of factors needs to be considered, leaders 'legitimate doubt'.[15] Leaders know that the journey always ends somewhere different from what was originally anticipated and the route is full of unforeseen difficulties. Having clarified where people think they are going, and why, leaders encourage them to explore new options with an open and optimistic mind. This often helps people to discover that what they thought they knew was not so certain after all.

As a general practitioner (GP) I find it helpful to move between a focus on named threats and a broad exploration of uncertainty. I find myself very preoccupied with failure when I see a child who might have early meningitis. However, in most consultations I am preoccupied with listening carefully, and opening the conversation out to get beyond the immediate presenting complaint to understand a breadth of things that matter.

Weick's distinction is the same one I make between linear and systems thinking. Immediate, clear threats require clear, decisive action. In these situations leaders, managers and facilitators fulfil traditional roles of making decisions, achieving targets and facilitating processes.

More complex situations can be made worse by precipitous decisions. Instead they need systematic, thoughtful exploration of possibilities. Leaders, managers and facilitators all help people to move from places that seem certain (but probably are not), through uncertainty, to places that may or may not feel certain. Uncertainty is the one guaranteed feature. As Thompson puts it: 'Coping with uncertainty [is] the essence of the administrative process'.[16]

Leaders help people to be less fearful of uncertainty. They recognise that the more you know, the more you know you don't know. The certainty of destination is replaced by a concern that the journey is filled with possibilities. This idea encourages travellers to be alert to the extraordinary potential of the present moment, listening with all the senses to things that are said and unsaid, seen and unseen, and reflecting experiences against many other experiences to find new patterns and new questions to ask. Moss Kanter writes: 'How do you study the future? One way is by listening'.[17]

Wheatley and Kellner-Rogers maintain: 'Organization wants to happen. Human organizations emerge from processes that can be comprehended but never controlled'.[18]

The participation of fellow travellers helps all involved to comprehend the meaning inside a specific context. Burns describes how 'The chief executives of Oticon and PCI both wanted to transform their organisations. One gained the support of his colleagues and employees and succeeded, the other did not and failed'.[19]

Huber summarises lessons about leadership:

> The most important and recurrent lessons for managers [are]:
>
> 1 Even change, itself, is changing.
> 2 Organizational success and survival depend on continuous and discontinuous improvements.
> 3 Increasing volumes and varieties of information processing and analysis are the norm for successful organizations.
> 4 Teamwork and shared values are critical for managing change and enhancing organizational performance.[20]

These extracts from these giants in the theory of organisational behaviour suggest that leaders for integrated primary health care inevitably have to deal with situations that are complex and unpredictable. Leaders must 'listen to the whispers' as well as to the loud shouts, they must reflect on overall meaning as well as on discrete facts, facilitate participation as well as signpost clear direction and take risks about next steps that make sense inside a situation but defy understanding further away. Leaders often 'feel' as much as 'see' the best way forward, and bring together different forces to point things in the most optimistic direction.

These writers do not always use the word 'leader'. This kind of leadership goes by many names: managers, systems practitioners, facilitators . . .

Such leaders often 'lead from behind' – watching the backs of others as they take risks. This is the image of a parent who helps a child to learn by doing. As Bennis put it: 'The process of becoming a leader is much the same as the process of becoming an integrated human being.[21]

In the context of integrated primary health care I make no significant distinction between leaders, systems practitioners, managers, facilitators and mature citizens. All recognise that successful change is a journey into uncertainty, where multiple factors interact and adapt to each other. All are concerned with how individual journeys can make sense to complex social travel. All have an optimistic and listening approach that helps people to travel hopefully.

The author's story

I was primary care facilitator in Liverpool for five years from 1989. Before then I had been a GP in the city. Liverpool is one of the most deprived cities in Europe and general practice development had previously been neglected. I was suspicious that initiatives that developed general practice in isolation from other disciplines would not suffice, so I worked as part of a multi-disciplinary facilitation team to develop the whole primary care community. We used a broad understanding of primary health care and related closely to the Liverpool Healthy City 2000 Project. The first team included a nurse, a practice manager and myself. We sent regular interactive bulletins (monthly at first) to all GPs in the 110 practices in the city, asking what they considered to be the priorities for our work. We included a summary of their replies in subsequent bulletins in order to produce an ongoing conversation throughout primary care that identified priorities, facilitated coordinated action, fed back progress and identified new concerns. A senior management group facilitated integration of institutional policy and a multi-disciplinary support group facilitated local collaborations. Both evaluated progress.

In 1989 the employment of practice nurses emerged as the biggest priority. We facilitated an open meeting attended by GPs and nurses from politics, academia and everyday practice, and health authority managers. We structured the meeting so that different perspectives could be aired and challenged in small and large groups. Agreements about what should be done were marked in plenary sessions. The facilitation team subsequently helped the partner agencies to complete their action plans, devise model job descriptions, develop interviewing skills, write university courses, and analyse pay, training and professional issues. We used the interactive bulletins to keep these issues alive while also doing pilot work to deal with other concerns.

Between 1989 and 1991 this approach produced a proliferation of innovation, described by the then professor of general practice as a 'bush fire'. Lay health workers helped practices to make their waiting rooms places where people could learn. A diary for all health workers provided useful information. The number of employed practice nurses increased from eight to 110, covering almost every practice. A new university practice nurse course started. The first practice nurse mentor scheme in the UK started, and a training course in facilitation skills was devised for them. Health promotion clinics developed in virtually every practice. Practice nurses started to lead in-practice multi-disciplinary workshops and cross-practice multi-disciplinary locality learning. By 1993, multi-disciplinary teams of facilitators were helping clusters of about 20 practices to develop local collaborations for health. The immunisation and cervical cytology rates in the areas we targeted soared.

People hardly seemed to notice. Everyone (rightly) considered that they had done it themselves. We had no theory at that time to explain whole-system change. Shared purpose had developed between everyone involved, and they had spontaneously devised projects to test next steps. Ongoing feedback enabled ongoing adaptation. The achievements were unexpectedly great, and they seemed to happen by magic.

An unpleasant surprise

Immediately after the increase in practice nurse employment a group of GPs challenged us, stating that we had done a lot for nurses but nothing for them. This was an unconvincing argument because it was they who had asked us to prioritise nurse employment.

This anecdote signals a common and powerful force that works against integrated primary health care. I have witnessed a similar challenge on many occasions, from different disciplines and in different contexts. On each occasion I perceive challengers who strongly identify with linear notions of change, and after they had experienced success from a set of multi-disciplinary interventions that they had invited or commissioned, and which had a greater effect than they expected. In each instance they made allegations that did not stand scrutiny, but they also disallowed scrutiny. They chose situations where the accused had no chance to defend themselves. Most curious of all there was no apparent gain to them from doing this.

Pause

How have you made sense of experiences like this when they have happened to you?

The need for better theory

To highlight the Liverpool anecdote is an unfair distortion of some remarkable years. The conflict I am describing manifested itself in one meeting and many of the people involved later became firm friends. But it is the clearest example I have of an important message of this book – when people do not have an adequate explanatory model of whole-system change they obstruct it. In particular, medical practitioners overly expect the world to behave in linear ways and this limits their constructive involvement in integrated primary health care (Chapter 9), even though GPs are natural leaders of it (Chapter 10).

To understand this phenomenon better, here, I wish to start a discussion about power, identity and culture. I want to persuade you that this defensive behaviour is understandable, normal and even desirable. I continue this discussion in chapters 12 and 13.

One interpretation of my anecdote is that our team challenged the power of the people concerned. I shall start with a discussion of power.

Power is present at all levels and stages of change of organisational change. Morgan describes 14 sources of power in organisations.[22] Yet the significance of power is rarely acknowledged in health service language, and it is often trivialised through throw-away references to 'carrots and sticks'. A much fuller understanding of power is needed.

Lukes states: 'to have power is to be able to make a difference to the world . . . Those interested in power are interested in two things: in the difference that is made and in the making of that difference'.[23]

By this definition my teams and I clearly had power – significant differences happened as a result of our interventions. But what form of power? Some of it was Arendt's notion of the 'power of persuasion' that shapes a consensus.[24] But we were much more pro-active than is implied in this notion of power as 'influence'. We used every available lever for change; we pushed and pulled, argued, modelled and supported. In particular, we helped different people to find common purpose and align their interests. Wherever we found energy for change we supported it, and helped the enthusiasts to point their work to the work of others. It was a multi-faceted, non-linear form of power that enlivened things throughout the whole system. It set up a dynamic between different players that stimulated creative interactions. This is the form of power described by Foucault as 'productive power' that 'has multiple effects, constitutive as well as destructive, facilitative as well as coercive . . . not a resource concentrated in the hands of a few, but multiply sourced and heterogeneous in its effects.[25]

By contrast, the responses we experienced involved a linear form of power – the Marx/Dahl/Weber notion of power as domination: 'which permits the more powerful agents to control, coerce or induce the less powerful agents to do their bidding'.[25]

This analysis helps to recognise that recognisable forms of power were at play. But I find it implausible to explain the conflict as a challenge to the GPs' power. It was their power that gave rise to this successful project and it achieved what the GPs said they wanted. They had the power to fashion the next steps. Subsequent behaviour was supportive. If anything, their power was enhanced.

So why did these people behave in this way? Why such a brutal response to success that they had asked for? Why no preparedness to discuss the issues? This is extremely defensive behaviour.

Personal constructs and mental models

Kelly's personal construct theory offers an explanation. He maintained that all people 'develop belief systems about how the world operates. They test out the validity of these belief systems through behavioural experiments . . . the degree to which constructs change is determined by their permeability'.[26]

An interpretation I prefer is that our approach challenged the GPs' belief system about how the world behaves, and this felt like an attack on their very sense of self and authority. The challengers expected the world to behave in a simple and predictable way. They had insufficient 'permeability' – insufficient exposure to, and understanding of, alternative explanations. What we did, by their expectation, was impossible. It felt like magic. The GPs found themselves in a new multi-disciplinary team and did not know how to behave within it. The whole thing left them feeling exposed, confused and defensive.

I find this more plausible because I did not perceive malicious intent. I saw panic. I do not believe the GPs meant harm. Instead, I believe that they felt that things were out of control as they understood 'control'. Control, as they knew it, was a linear direct form.

It is easy to see where this linear construct comes from in the case of medics. Medical students are at the top of the class at school. We learn a combative approach to disease cure, and largely appeal to a reductionist science to justify our actions. We learn in uni-disciplinary groups, divorced from the real world of multiple interactions and ongoing complex change. Of course this leads to a linear mindset – where else would it lead?

The question facing a student of leadership is: can this be changed? My experience says it can – exposure to multi-disciplinary team-working and theories about non-linearity can develop more flexible constructs with which to understand a complex interactive world. And this is what happened, for there is a postscript to the Liverpool story.

Within days of that heated meeting some of the same doctors became more involved. Within months many started to promote our work. Two years later the group as a whole apologised, and many became strong advocates of multi-disciplinary, team-oriented, integrated primary health care. With hindsight, that meeting may even have been a catalyst for their greater participation.

I had the opportunity some years later to discuss with a key person what the conflict was all about from the GPs' point of view. He explained to me that the GPs could not make sense of what was happening. They were too far out of their comfort zones. He said, with an understanding smile: 'We would have got there in the end – but it might have taken us 20 years.'

Alinsky observed a similar phenomenon which arises when things happen that are outside of people's expectations. He tried to give away $10 notes to people in the street and experienced blunt rejection from everyone he approached.[27]

Linear and systems thinking are incompatible unless . . .

In chapters 12 and 13 I shall argue that 'linear thinking' is not a fault particularly of medics – it is a necessary way of thinking of all human beings to retain a sense of personal coherence (along with other necessary non-linear ways of thinking).

Linear thinking dominates theories of science, health and change. It is the idea that the world is 'naturally' ordered into discrete unchanging particles which affect each other in direct and predictable ways, like hitting a billiard ball. In the 'real world' multiple billiard balls interact, and each ball is itself undergoing ongoing change, making the billiard ball image misleading.

Linear thinking is particularly useful when short-term priorities and hierarchical, individualistic values dominate. It is a common defence mechanism in those who feel uncertain about themselves – perhaps threatened or vulnerable. But as a sole philosophy it promotes blaming, avoidance and stereotyping rather than listening, reflection and change. It produces withdrawal rather than engagement. It results in a reactive and short-term, 'reductionist' approach to planning and the poor performance of teams.

By contrast, 'systems thinking' recognises that everything connects. It encourages listening to, and understanding, other people's point of view, finding long-term solutions, seeing bigger pictures. Nevertheless, as a sole philosophy it also has disadvantages, promoting time-consuming exploration of difference, unproductive circular talk and indecisive action. Integrated primary health care needs practitioners, managers and citizens to be able to think in both linear *and* systems ways. They need to be skilled at switching from one to the other to find the combination appropriate for the moment.

But there is a paradox here that will lead to lose–lose outcomes unless resolved: linear thinkers cannot achieve what they want without a systems approach – but their philosophy does not allow a systems ways of thinking to exist.

By contrast, systems thinking can accommodate linear thinking as one focus within a bigger picture. It can transcend but include linear thinking. In Part III I suggest that repeatedly moving between focused detail and bigger pictures is the way to resolve this paradox to produce win–win ways forward.

The distinction between linear and systems thinking is witnessed in a railway system. Trains undertake linear journeys along named lines to discrete stations. All of these are previously agreed and predictable. By contrast, travellers choose destinations which are meaningful to them. They choose discrete trains, lines and stations to use as part of a bigger quest that is their own life story (Chapter 12). Railways need linear thinking to provide an efficient railway network. Travellers need systems thinking to decide their journeys. Trains without travellers are meaningless. They are inter-dependent, but different. Both are needed.

In parts II and IV I describe practical ways to help people to make linear thinking and systems thinking relevant to each other.

Bird's nest belief system

> **Pause**
>
> *What theories do you find useful to understand the behaviour of people in complex uncertain situations?*

In all parts of this book I try to bring real-life experience to a discussion of theory. Central to my argument is that experience is more complex than any words can describe. We have to use words because they are a main mechanism to communicate ideas. But they can never do justice to the full experience. I explore the limitation of words and theories in Chapter 11, where I argue that the dominant understanding of scientific knowledge (linear, quantitative, positivist) can be made relevant to complex changing situations by also simultaneously using two complementary theories of knowledge, termed 'critical theory' and 'constructivism'. These lead to qualitative and participatory approaches to enquiry.

Experience is gained through interaction in the world. It is a main mechanism whereby we create and change our identities and life stories, our habits and webs of relationships. Through experience we develop our personal constructs – mental models, theories and motivations.

Leavey offers a more complex understanding of personal constructs. He argues that people are capable of thinking in many different and paradoxical ways. He describes how all people pick ideas about the world from here and there, to describe a cluster of beliefs that they use in different circumstances. He calls it their 'bird's nest belief systems'[28] – the cluster of beliefs that 'feather the nest' that is their identity.

Leavey helps us to recognise that people do not have to think solely with one main mental model. An array of mental models can co-exist. People can use different ones from a menu of options, depending on the effect they want to have and also depending on having them in the 'nest' to begin with.

Towards a theory of whole-system learning and change

We do not have to divide the world into linear thinkers and systems thinkers. Instead, people have the ability to move between one and the other mindset, appropriately for the context. And this is what happens in real life – when that bus is bearing down on you, you quickly switch into a linear mindset and jump out of the way. When you are tending a garden you quickly learn that different plants like different amounts of light. This complex mental adaptation to the specific needs of a context is what is called 'common sense'.

The central issue here is not the desirability of combining linear and systems thinking, nor people's ability to move between them. The central issue is that we are largely expected by academics and practitioners alike to use linear theories of how the world works. To deal with real situations we need to move between different ways of thinking.

In Chapter 13 I relate the conflict between linear and systems thinking to the claim by Argyris and Schon that hidden 'theories-in-use' (the mental models which underpin what people do rather than what they say) subvert most attempts at change, and are undiscussable:[10] you aren't even allowed to talk about them. I argue that movement between them can result in a changed sense of self which results in changed behaviour.

Also in Chapter 13 I propose a set of practical policies to help people to learn in this broader and deeper way. These policies will help to develop a community culture which values diversity and holistic thinking, helps individuals to self-organise and to lead collaboration and helps people to see the multiple influences that affect change, attributing success appropriately.

Through lack of adequate theory our Liverpool facilitation teams repeatedly experienced misattribution of our work, almost exclusively from those who did not actually take part in it. We facilitated a successful six-month intervention to improve relations in an unhappy health centre – success was later attributed to a new building. We facilitated a successful two-year intervention to develop multi-disciplinary reflection and enquiry in a network of practices in a deprived outer estate – success was later attributed to a part-time young GP employed in one of the practices. People on the ground knew that these were not true, but none of us had at that time an alternative theory to offer.

Our teams continued to apply the same principles of whole-system learning in many other projects: in teambuilding workshops for general practices; in health promotion initiatives where lay workers worked in the waiting rooms of half the general practices in the city; in a cross-city coalition for heart disease prevention involving the City Council and trade unions as well as health, business, learning and voluntary sectors. In every case, unexpected and significant things resulted. Those involved were proud of the improvements to quality they had made.

I now recognise that we provided an ongoing and visible infrastructure of communication and facilitation which helped people to see how their work could be relevant to bigger stories. Through inter-disciplinary learning and enquiry, and participatory whole-system events, we helped stakeholders throughout the whole system to recognise how they could change in complementary ways. Coalitions of interest led different aspects of change, and progress was fed back at agreed times to witness the whole evolving picture, provoking further learning and adaptation. We adopted the principles of a learning organisation as described by Senge,[6] and a learning community, as described by Wenger.[29] We advocated the pillars of primary health care, as analysed by Macdonald.[30] We facilitated whole-system change through a process of 'incremental revolution', as observed by McNulty and Ferlie.[31] I did not know this then. All I knew was that it worked.

In this book I wish to set down what I have learnt – practically in parts II and IV, and theoretically in parts I and III. This is not magic. It is the understandable behaviour of human beings when offered the chance to take steps through uncertainty, from which they enhance their own sense of identity and, at the same time, contribute to a more caring society. Leadership helps them to take these steps and see the bigger stories in which they are walking.

References

1 Kolb D (1984) *Experiential Learning*. Prentice Hall, Englewood Cliffs, NJ.
2 Schon DA (1983) *The Reflective Practitioner*. Maurice Temple Smith, London.
3 Revans R (1998) *ABC of Action Learning*. Lemos & Crane, London.
4 Whyte WF (1991) *Participatory Action Research*. Sage, New York, NY.
5 Ison R and Russell D (2000) *Agricultural Extension and Rural Development*. Cambridge University Press, Cambridge.
6 Senge P (1993) *The Fifth Discipline*. Century Hutchinson, London.
7 Wenger E (2000) Communities of practice and social learning systems. *Organization*. 7: 225–46.
8 Whitney D and Trosten-Bloom A (2003) *The Power of Appreciative Inquiry*. Berrett-Koehler, San Francisco, CA.
9 Cooperrider DL, Sorenson PF Jnr, Yeager TF and Whitney D. (2001) *Appreciative Inquiry: an emerging direction for organizational development*. Stipes, Champaign, IL.
10 Argyris C and Schon DA (1996) *Organizational Learning 2 – Theory, Method, and Practice*. Addison Wesley, Reading, MA.
11 Sadler P (2003) *Leadership*. Kogan Page, London.

12 Jackson N (2003) Introduction to brokering in higher education. In: N Jackson (ed) *Engaging and Changing Higher Education Through Brokerage*. Ashgate Publishing, Aldershot.

13 Weick KE (1995) *Sensemaking in Organizations*. Sage, Thousand Oaks, CA.

14 Weick KE (2001) *Managing the Unexpected – Assuring High Performance in an Age of Complexity*. Sage, Thousand Oaks, CA.

15 Weick KE (2001) Leadership as the legitimization of doubt. In: W Bennis, GM Spreitzer and T Cummings (eds). *The Future of Leadership: today's top leadership thinkers speak to tomorrow's leaders*. Jossey-Bass, San Francisco, CA.

16 Thompson JD (1967) *Organizations in Action. Social Science Basis of Administration Theory*. McGraw Hill, New York, NY.

17 Moss Kanter R (1989) *When Giants Learn to Dance*. Thomson Business Press, London.

18 Wheatley M and Kellner-Rogers M (1996) *A Simpler Way*. Berrett-Koehler, San Francisco, CA.

19 Burnes B (1996) *Managing Change – A Strategic Approach to Organisational Dynamics*. Pitman Publishing, St Ives.

20 Huber GP and Glick WH (1996) What was learned about organizational change and redesign. In: GP Huber and WH Glick (eds) *Organizational Change and Redesign*. Oxford University Press, Oxford.

21 Bennis W and Goldsmith J (2003) *Learning to Lead: a workbook on becoming a leader*. Basic Books, New York, NY.

22 Morgan G (1997) *Images of Organization*. Sage, Thousand Oaks, CA.

23 Lukes S (2005) Introduction. In: S Lukes (ed) *Power: Readings in Social and Political Theory, No. 4*. New York University Press, New York, NY.

24 Arendt H (1986) Communicative power. In: S Lukes (ed) *Power: Readings in Social and Political Theory, No. 4*. New York University Press, New York, NY.

25 Ashcroft RE (2005) Power, corruption and lies: ethics and power. In: RE Ashcroft, MG Parker, M Verkerk, G Widdershoven and AM Lucassen (eds) *Case Analysis in Clinical Ethics*. Cambridge University Press, Cambridge.

26 Carr A (2000) Theories that focus on belief systems. In: A Carr (ed) *Family Therapy. Concepts, Processes and Practice*. John Wiley, London.

27 Alinski SD (1972) *Rules for Radicals*. Vintage Books, New York, NY.

28 Leavey C (2000) *Why do women not attend for cervical smear appointments?* (dissertation). Centre for Health, Healing and Human Development, Liverpool John Moores University.

29 Wenger E (1998) *Communities of Practice – Learning, Meaning, Identity*. Cambridge University Press, Cambridge.

30 Macdonald JJ (1992) *Primary Health Care – Medicine in its Place*. Earthscan Publications, London.

31 McNulty T and Ferlie E (2002) *Reengineering Health Care – The Complexities of Organizational Transformation*. Oxford University Press, Oxford.

Chapter 2

New ways of thinking about leadership

Summary

Individual heroic leaders are not enough to develop integrated primary health care. 'Shared leadership' is a useful idea when considering learning and change throughout a whole system. It is a form of advanced team-working where the team as a whole has a leadership role, and also individual team members have personal leadership roles for different constituencies. This broader understanding of leadership is needed at all levels of society for integrated primary health care to become a reality.

The theory and language of this notion of leadership are poorly developed. But it is evidenced all the time, going by whatever language is acceptable in each context: 'patients-as-partners', 'team-working', 'family and community development', 'strategic coalitions' and 'networks'.

In each of these languages the focus is on the interconnecting forces, which are invisible at a distance but are very real when you are involved, and the main thing that makes things work (or not). Leaders recognise that all people are connected in webs of relationships that can constrain or enable change.

Individual leaders and shared leadership alike help people from the constituencies served to take calculated risks in complex and uncertain situations. They help them to find ways forwards which make sense to them and also to the system as a whole.

Leadership for whole-system learning and change frees up creative thinking by enabling learning between people who have different insights. Leaders need an infrastructure of communication and facilitation to sense the winds of change, solve crises and facilitate cross-organisation innovation.

Leaders make sure that there are regular points where learning is fed back to all stakeholders and next steps are agreed. This produces a 'whole-system conversation'.

Leaders help people to self-organise in ways that surface their mental models and hidden motivations. This produces coalitions of interest whose members know each other at more than superficial levels.

Leaders combine the energies of diverse motivated groups with a variety of other forces to produce momentum for whole-system change.

The image of interactive jugglers (see Figure 2.1) shows that integration requires changes in the behaviour of all concerned. Interactive juggling is a process of team development which requires patient rehearsal of passing objects between the players. The players can become high-performing teams with intuitive understanding of their potential as a whole, and the skills to achieve this. The model of a leader entering and exiting a system shows that boundaries are necessary and temporary structures which allow focused work to take place within much greater complexity.

Leadership is often thought to be solely the role of an exceptional individual – a knight in shining armour who bravely leads followers onwards in one direction. This image blinds us to the reality that a named leader is merely the most obvious person from a team – or from several teams. It also blinds us to the idea that sustainable change requires different people to travel in different but complementary directions. Integrated primary health care needs leadership for each of these journeys and shared leadership which integrates many journeys.

In Chapter 1 I explained that leadership for integrated primary health care is concerned less with a linear notion of leaders-and-followers and more with making sense of complex whole stories. Leaders may still think and act in controlling ways, but they will be equally concerned with helping people to think for themselves, and to produce complementary changes in different organisations and disciplines, creating new relationships and behaviours.

Shared leadership[1] is a helpful idea when considering multiple complementary changes that help whole systems to change. This is an advanced form of team-working where a multi-disciplinary group as a whole has a leadership role, and individual team members have complementary personal leadership roles. This image permits each to be a hero at the appropriate time. It also allows the more common and less glamorous notion that leadership helps people of different backgrounds to make sense of proposed changes, and empowers them to do complementary things in a shared effort for learning and change.

The theory and language of this notion of leadership is poorly developed, but it is happening all the time, going by whatever language is acceptable in each context: 'patients-as-partners', 'team-working', 'family and community development', 'strategic coalitions' and 'networks'.

In each of these languages the focus is on the interconnecting forces, which are invisible at a distance but are extremely real when you are involved, and often the main thing that makes things work (or not). Leaders recognise that all people are connected in webs of relationships that can constrain or enable change.

In this chapter I offer a set of ideas to illuminate this new notion of leadership. No one idea conveys it all. Each looks at it from a different angle to build up a richer picture of something that can actually only be understood when you do it.

Leaders help stories to unfold

Pause

Do you know someone whom you call a good leader who has not influenced the evolution of an important story?

It is not specific learning that preoccupies leaders, but moving forward the whole story. Almost always leaders encounter change halfway through a story in which many mistakes have already been made. Leaders help individuals and groups to move from this sense of chaos to a place where things seem coherent. Leaders hold the story even when others have 'lost the plot'.

Leaders create learning spaces

Leaders are skilled at creating places where people of different backgrounds learn from and with each other. Some decide to develop shared projects, through which the participants develop relationships for future collaborations.

In learning spaces people tell their stories (Chapter 12) and highlight the things that are meaningful to them. They describe their shared view about the way things should be. Techniques such as games and role-play (Chapter 17) can surface deeper motivations about which the individuals themselves are unaware. A learning space helps to mix and match different interests and obligations to form teams with a shared need.

Leadership helps three different types of learning

Leaders help people to ask questions which will move them forwards at the edge of their comfort zones (too easy and they don't learn, too hard and they disengage). Different types of question lead to different types of learning, as described by Argyris and Schon.[2]

- 'Single-loop learning'[2] asks questions about what is known, checking out facts and looking for errors without challenging existing values or work practices. You may ask 'What is on the table?' and count the various things, or 'What would happen to my backache if I positioned my chair differently at the table?' Then it gathers data to answer the question. In single-loop learning the feedback loop leads back to confirm the original idea or plan, which is not expected to change significantly. An example is a quantitative audit that compares measures against standards of blood pressure control.
- By contrast, changing the form of something (transformational change) requires 'double-loop learning'.[2] Rather than asking what is on the table, you may ask 'What alternatives are there to tables?', or 'What set of things will help my long-term back problem?' The feedback loop of double-loop learning goes to another, as yet uncertain, place. The process challenges existing assumptions, including values and work practices. It explores new ways of doing things and potentially valuable new relationships. An example is a qualitative audit that asks patients which consulting approach helps them to relax when having their blood pressure taken.
- True innovation requires a third kind of learning: 'deutero-learning'.[2] This is a dynamic and participatory process of interaction between different ideas to find new and imaginative connections. This is the buzz of a focus group or a whole-system event. An example is a participatory audit where a general practice team and patients together consider new ways to provide integrated care for people with hypertension.

In Chapter 11 I relate these three types of learning to three theories of knowledge, termed positivism, critical theory and constructivism. I discuss their relevance to 'learning communities' in Chapter 13. Leadership uses all three kinds of learning to get beyond superficial words of agreement to work together and achieve genuine changes in the relationships and work practices of people throughout a whole system.

Leaders reduce uncertainty

Leaders reduce uncertainty in seemingly chaotic situations by clarifying what is known and what is not. They do this by giving space for all involved to have their perspectives heard, clarifying what they have agreed together and what general direction makes sense to the group as a whole. This is single-loop learning – clarifying what is agreed, or known (and what is not).

Leaders legitimate doubt[3]

Leadership also helps people to take tentative steps into the unknown. This is double-loop learning – exploring the unknown. Leaders help people to realise that they do not have to know everything and it is OK to make certain mistakes – as long as they learn from them and change as a result.

Leaders develop mechanisms for ongoing communication and mutual learning

Leaders recognise that individuals and groups will misunderstand others and create conflicts if they feel that they are on opposite sides. Agreed times for ongoing communication and mutual learning helps to develop a sense of unity. This must help different points of view to be truly heard, and trusted relationships to be built. Thinking laterally about how various views can enhance each other results in new knowledge and new ways forward. This is the dynamic process of deutero-learning – finding new and imaginative connections between different people's insights that can lead to innovation.

Leaders build an infrastructure of facilitation and communication

Pause

Do you know someone whom you call a good leader who has not built systems of communication?

Everything is changing constantly. If something appears to be static it is merely changing slowly. To cope with this movement, leaders create networks of people who can sense the winds of change and can convene the right kind of groups to think through what to do about them. Both in times of crisis and as a routine procedure, these people feed back ideas about future direction. Leaders complete the cycle by feeding back to them information that is amalgamated from different places. This creates an ongoing 'whole-system conversation'.

Many people within a network are already leaders, in that they motivate others to relate their work to an integrated picture of health. Leadership involves releasing the potential of these people to work as teams which connect different organisations. Networks of networks can make it easier for different leadership teams to collaborate. Each team produces incremental progress. Leadership helps these to connect to have a bigger, cultural-changing effect.

Leaders think and act strategically

Leaders avoid running here and there, and reacting to the latest crisis with noise. Instead, they anticipate different kinds of problems and get people within their networks thinking about how to respond to them before they come to a head. They use crises as opportunities to develop leaders. They create the future rather than jump to the past. They bring into view things that are essential for success but are initially invisible. They make a sharp distinction between a strategy that will work, and the language needed to sell the idea to different stakeholders.

Being ahead of problems in this way requires predictable places where various teams come together to revisit their shared vision and redesign the plans in the light of new events. It demands techniques which map the complexities involved and help people to grapple with them.

Like a general, linking troop movements and supply lines, leaders plan their networks and learning spaces to produce desired outcomes at desired times. Like a stage manager they get to know where the plate-spinners are and support them to spin better.

Leaders combine subtle and nurturing attitudes with a sharp analysis of which different constituencies, teams and goals are relevant at that phase of develop-ment. They are skilled at rapid appraisal that brings together different kinds of knowledge to reveal a rich picture.

Leaders handle complexity and simplicity with equal ease

Leaders distinguish between 'simple situations', which need a direct response, 'complicated situations', which need complicated system maps, and 'complex situations', which need facilitation of inter-agency learning and adaptation. Like the experienced car driver they may follow a simple, already-defined route. But they will also know how to navigate the back streets when the traffic news alerts them to congestion ahead. They observe the momentum of cars coming from different directions, and calculate what speed and direction they should choose. They also consider ways to improve the whole traffic industry, and identify which signposts will give people options for new routes.

Leaders create shared social space

Health care is full of bureaucracies. These are particularly poor at enabling innovation because they are full of linear structures. In bureaucracies, practi-tioners live in segregated boxes that fragment effort and have (vertical) 'line management'. This prevents (horizontal) learning from those who are different, and the development of relationships. It stifles innovation. Leaders facilitate playful interaction between people who are different. They do this by creating shared social space. This takes many forms: carnivals, parties, corner shops, churches, bars, schools, projects and everyday meetings.

Leaders are team players

A team of leaders is not any sort of team. The word *team* originates from farming – a team of oxen is harnessed to a plough and the reins are in the hands of a driver. This is not the image that facilitates learning and change in whole systems. A better image is that of a football team. In a successful football team individuals are so rehearsed in communication and understanding of each other's skills that they pass the ball in creative ways to gain advantage for the team as a whole.

Consider a poor football team, where individual players are unable to see beyond their own self-importance or do not know how to get the best out of other team members. It is in the good team that the brilliance of individuals can best be shown. The team which overly values individual talent over team performance is not even very good at showing off individual talent. In a football team the players can easily see each other on the pitch. They practise synchronous working day after day to learn how they can best succeed as a whole. Leadership for health care must similarly make it easy for people throughout the whole system to 'see' each other, rehearse co-ordinated activity and pause to reflect and learn.

Leaders remain balanced in the high seas

This idea of leadership is dynamic and dependent on trusted relationships. It recognises that multiple moving parts are connected in multiple overlapping wholes. Rather than expecting reality to be fixed into the ground, reality is balanced on rafts at sea. To go forwards you have to loosen your tight grip on the anchors that once felt so secure. Instead, you feel the multiple movements beneath your feet and use all your senses to feel the winds of change. Leadership is concerned with mastery rather than with control. If you are a good sailor/ leader, you can achieve mastery in your little boat, but you can never control all the elements.

Leaders facilitate synchrony between different forces for change

Pause
Do you know someone whom you call a good leader who has not enabled the coming together of different forces?

The ideas in this book start from the assumption that people are complex. Simple categorisations lead to unhelpful stereotyping: 'men think like this and women think like that'; 'blacks behave like this and whites behave like that'; 'she [he] is a natural leader'; 'only money will motivate people to change'. Even when there is some truth in such stereotypes there will be many other equally true insights into the behaviour of the same people. This simple stereotyping has little place in strategies for change because it does not give insight into the subtle and complex factors needed for different people to find common purpose and change things in harmony. These simplistic pre-judgements are *prejudices* – they lead to discrimination and inequity.

Having said this, leaders must also remember that people who have been subjected to persistent stereotyping, or, for that matter, any form of sustained misunderstanding or abuse, commonly exhibit defensive behaviour. This may manifest itself as stereotypic behaviour, but it should be seen largely as the consequence of the original insult, needing support and personal development, rather than further stereotyping.

Leadership recognises that people have multiple motivations, fears, defence mechanisms and potentials that are not evident at first sight (Chapter 12). Well-managed change takes people from wherever they are to places that are good both for them and for their communities. This requires that people clarify their shared vision, and create their own incremental steps towards it. Their own goals are therefore, in part, defined by their personal motivations. This means that local motivation can pull change forwards by its own interests, as well as being driven by forces beyond its control (thanks to Siobhan Clarke for the clarity of this point).

The skill of simultaneously driving and pulling change is only part of what leaders do to stimulate change. When inertia is high leaders may exaggerate external threats and stimulate crises to get people ready for action. When change is happening too fast leaders may dampen down enthusiasm. In both cases they are facilitating synchrony between different forces and motivating factors to create an environment in which reflection and action are more likely.

Sometimes leaders of integration are visionaries, able to see further than others; at other times they are neutral diplomats, concerned with finding common purpose between different groups. In both instances they are concerned with:

- coherent change that uses the motivations of stakeholders to move things forwards
- creating a sustainable infrastructure of feedback and review
- developing leadership skills among the stakeholders who will facilitate later progress.

These three things mark a difference from the traditional understanding of leadership, which has tended to emphasise driving change through the concerns of 'inconvenient' stakeholders, has prioritised short-term projects over sustainable development and has seen new leaders as a threat to their own authority.

An image: interactive jugglers

The image of this chapter is of jugglers interacting. I have adapted this image (Figure 2.1) from one used by the Open University Systems Unit. As a leader and as a citizen you will have to juggle your commitments and interact with other jugglers. You can make juggling fun and creative, or you can make it stressful – you have a degree of choice about this.

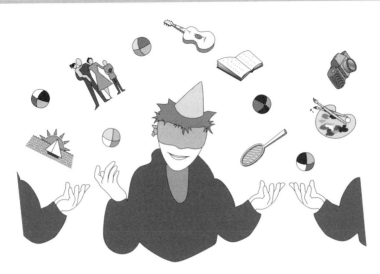

Figure 2.1 Interactive jugglers.

First, see what one juggler alone does. She knows where all the balls are, they are a manageable number and of similar size. If she does not know where they are, or if there are too many, they drop. If one ball is much bigger than the others, she stops juggling.

See what happens when there are two jugglers. They have different rhythms and juggle different kinds of things. Juggling between them is team-working. You can see why the phases of team development are necessary: 'norming', 'storming', 'forming', 'performing'. Norming is examining the ways in which the other juggles in preparation for a game of interactive juggling. Storming is when each wants the shared juggling to happen in their preferred style, and forming is when they find a mutually agreeable formula, which is probably a style new to both. Performing is the polished finished result presented to the outside world. High quality teamwork requires patient and sustained development. It does not become 'polished' until the later stages.

There is a final stage – mourning. There can be a big sense of loss when good teams end.

Leadership is concerned with developing the skills of both individual and shared juggling. There are large numbers of jugglers all over the place, juggling different things differently. They are largely unaware of each other, and are unaware they are doing things in incompatible ways. Leadership helps them to identify this and finds ways for them to relate better to each other. This, incrementally, transforms the whole system of which they are a part.

Pause

What interactive juggling do you do and how can you do it better?

A model: entering and exiting a system

The model shows 11 different stages within an intervention for change (Figure 2.2). Each stage requires you to do different things to be successful and to avoid pitfalls. Different parts of your work may be at different stages at the same time. The stages are not necessarily encountered in this order. I present them in this way to give a sense of progression through different stages and to show that different stages have different demands.

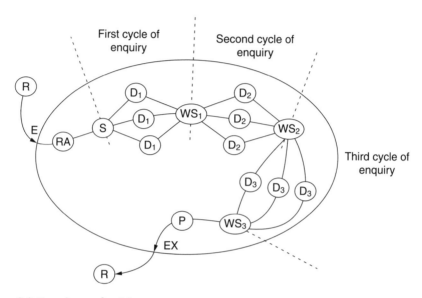

Figure 2.2 Entering and exiting a system. E = entry; RA = rapid appraisal; S = stakeholder consultation; D_1 = data gathering 1; WS_1 = whole-system event 1; D_2 = data gathering 2; WS_2 = whole-system event 2; DG_3 = data gathering 3; WS_3 = whole-system event 3; P = new policy; EX = exit; R = review.

The model shows a leader entering and exiting a situation in which he or she facilitates three cycles of reflection and action with stakeholders.

- The first cycle of enquiry helps participants to see what the present situation is, and to agree the rationale for change. This clarifies what is known and what is not. For example, a baseline audit may be needed, establishing data about workloads. The first cycle may also test if the vision people say they want is really what they want.
- The second cycle of enquiry contributes several different kinds of insight into what might be. This gives participants space to be creative, to act on their instincts in devising new programmes of work and to gather data about what happens. For example, different teams could undertake small projects, or analyse what has been done in other places.
- The third cycle of enquiry creates policy for new ways to do things which draws on insights from the previous stages and from the experiences of participants.

Three connected cycles provide opportunities to solve unforeseen problems with new ways of doing things, and also to examine unexpected consequences – good and bad. This provides a balanced view about whether the innovation really is a good thing.

These cycles can also start to build the infrastructure and leadership to sustain progress. By exiting at the end of the third cycle of enquiry the leader avoids dependency and signals to others their need to step into leadership roles. A new set of cycles can start straight away, but if there is no break at all people can become overwhelmed.

These cycles of reflection and inquiry can be called 'audits'. One advantage of this is that audit is an established professional responsibility. Senior colleagues will support it. Existing systems of support and monitoring can be refocused to support this activity. Summaries of individual and organisational audits can be collected together to provide a history of the development of the whole organisation.

Eleven different stages in an intervention for change

- **Entry (E).** You enter a new situation, or a new stage of an old situation. You will already have done preparatory work to establish if you want to enter or not. You will ask for a support or steering group to be set up that includes powerful people from the system of concern. This is a 'system transformation team' because it is charged with overseeing the transformation of the whole system, beyond your involvement. It will include representatives of the organisations and disciplines involved. It holds some authority of the whole system of concern. It is charged with protecting you from harm and building from your success. With this group you agree ground rules, roles and responsibilities.
- **Rapid appraisal (RA).** You undertake a rapid appraisal to map the stakeholders and understand their stories. This identifies different kinds of power in the system, and energy for change. It reveals an initial sense of what is achievable, and what the whole system of concern really is, rather than what it seemed to be at first sight. You put this analysis to the steering group and agree with them a way forward in which they all have roles.
- **Stakeholder consultation (S).** You facilitate discussions between stakeholders to understand which things matter to them and what are their future hopes. You list their concerns and gain their agreement for future involvement. You can do this within a whole-system event, at meetings of representatives, or through the post or by e-mail. This list gives rise to a set of agreements, goals and questions. Some of the questions frame the first cycle of enquiry, which is concerned largely with establishing what is the present state of affairs.
- **Data gathering 1 (D_1).** You may do this alone or with project teams. Your aim is to amalgamate baseline information, which illuminates the story so far and its future potential, mindful of the issues raised by the stakeholders. For example, you might want data on morbidity rates, or the achievement of targets, or details of forthcoming plans.
- **Whole-system event 1 (WS_1).** This is the first gathering of stakeholders to seriously consider the potential for change of the whole system of which they are a part. As with all whole-system events, leaders (perhaps you) first explain

the purpose of the meeting and summarise the story so far. In small groups participants describe to each other what things they value about the way things are and the future they hope to create. Participants consider the information they are given in the light of their own experiences and suggest a number of possible next steps. The whole conference chooses a set of priorities.

Many techniques can be used, such as brainstorming and diagramming, to map the system of concern (Chapter 14) and visualisation, fish bowl and role-play to gain different perspectives on things (Chapter 17). The design of whole-system events benefits from a backwards mapping approach (Chapter 6). Specific whole-system models are available (Chapter 15).

The event completes the first cycle of enquiry and starts the second. Participants consider which set of projects or questions will illuminate the next cycle, and project teams are agreed to lead these. The dates of the next two whole system events are agreed.

- **Data gathering 2 (D$_2$).** The project teams establish working relationships, gather data, lead a set of projects or enquiries and build their networks. They can be conceptualised as 'system redesign teams' since they are charged with undertaking stand-alone enquiries or projects, with a mind to how the insights they gain can contribute to redesign their part of a whole system.
- **Whole-system event 2 (WS$_2$).** This completes the second cycle of enquiry and starts the third. The project teams take significant roles at this event, both in planning and facilitating. Successes in their work are described, and lessons from them are considered in small groups. Through small-group–large-group iterations the whole conference comes to agree fruitful areas where cross-organisational teams could provide a shared leadership role, building both from the recent projects or evidence and other existing roles.

If things have progressed well (and this cannot be assumed) now is the time to start considering what long-term infrastructure will sustain longer-term communication. The steering group may need to be reconfigured to include perspectives previously not recognised to be important. The project teams may also need to be reformed.

Inadequate communication systems, overstretched or underdeveloped individuals can be temporarily moved sideways to develop away from the spotlight. Poorly functioning teams may need to be examined and strengthened. They may be part of the infrastructure for future sustainability and need to be developed in readiness for this role.

- **Data gathering 3 (D$_3$).** The project teams become more confident in this stage. They have become aware of their co-dependence on other teams and often spontaneously retain communication with them. They become increasingly able to see an emerging new shape and the practical implications of a new way of doing things. They become more able to represent the perspectives of their constituencies and sense what are realistic goals. They see obstacles before they arrive, and spot new potential quickly.

It is likely that the steering group will become more aware of its role in developing policy to support long-term successes. The group may start to value successes more, and critique them more thoughtfully. They may develop complementary cross-portfolio changes at a more central level to support sustainability of the changes that are appearing. Enquiry at this stage is concerned with exploring how to sustain progress and facilitate ongoing inter-organisational communication and facilitation. Several project teams may co-ordinate their work, gathering increasingly relevant data. The steering group may actively diverts resources to support these and be vocal about success.

- **Whole-system event 3 (WS$_3$).** This completes the third cycle of enquiry. It includes feedback about progress so far and agreement about policy within different organisations, which is, by now, not contentious. New roles, new system maps and new targets are agreed.
- **New policy (P).** New organisational policy signals the end of the sequence. In this area of concern things can now bed down. The organisations may certainly want more meetings, but a pause for breath before starting another is often the best thing.
- **Exit (EX).** This is a good time for you to move on to other things, or to negotiate a new role in a new stage of development. There are several reasons why this is helpful. If you, as leader, stay too long you can prevent others from moving to higher levels of responsibility. You can become overly equated with the success, or with a particular problem encountered somewhere along the way and prevent others from seeing the processes that underpin change. You can become too much of a force in your own right, and stifle further developments. You can become typecast as someone who only wants to be at the centre of controversy. You can become increasingly marginalised when no one knows how to nurture you or help you into different roles. Even if you stay, the process of exiting and re-entering is valuable for you and others to review your relationships.
- **Review life story (R).** When you leave a substantial piece of work it helps to reflect on what you have learnt about yourself and where you are going, before diving straight back in. Redraw your life-line (Chapter 14). Does it seem coherent to you? Do you need a mentor, or to undertake some personal exercises of self-exploration? Be careful not to confuse your sense of loss for loss of direction or motivation. You may be in a necessary stage of transition. Energy and insight will return when this is over.

The three cycles can take days, weeks or years to complete, and can involve multiple steps inbetween. The stages may not happen in the order listed. Sometimes getting people to the first whole-system event can take more time than everything else together. The complexity of the system to be developed has an important effect – changing a general practice system for repeat prescribing is of a different order to changing the system for care of the elderly across a city. But the principles are the same – a new system has to be built by those who will use it. It is built from patient, persistent cycles of reflection and action, testing new ways to do thing that develop trusted relations between the stakeholders. It is helpful to bunch the cycles of enquiry and action to maintain momentum and avoid overload – I find that three is good.

Three connected cycles also help participants to believe in the power of ongoing collective learning and action. The first cycle can be energising and productive, but few people will believe that things will follow through. When the second and third cycles have the same energising and productive effect people start to trust the process. If you stop before the third cycle the momentum can become lost.

References

1 Pearce CL and Conger JA (2003) *Shared Leadership – Reframing the Hows and Whys of Leadership*. Sage, Thousand Oaks, CA.
2 Argyris C and Schon DA (1996) *Organizational Learning 2 – Theory, Method, and Practice*. Addison Wesley, Reading, MA.
3 Weick KE. Leadership as the legitimisation of doubt. In: W Bennis, GM Spreitzer and T Cummings (eds) *The Future of Leadership: today's top leadership thinkers speak to tomorrow's leaders*. Jossey-Bass, San Francisco, CA.

Chapter 3

The extraordinary potential of primary care organisations

Summary

This chapter describes the organisational roles needed to achieve integrated primary health care, at the same time as dealing with the nuts and bolts of daily work that is, by its nature, reactive and short-term.

The World Health Organization (WHO) found huge obstacles to achieving integration when it tried, and failed, to operationalise the idea of comprehensive primary health care after the Alma Ata conference of 1978 (Chapter 9). Power, mismatch between needs and wants, and inadequate theory of organisations and systems are not the only obstacles. Different understandings of science, health and change mean that people aim for different things, use the same words to mean different things and say things they do not mean.

Primary care trusts (PCTs) came into being in 2003 in England. In other parts of the UK they are termed 'primary care organisations' (PCOs). They are large network-like institutions which took over some of the functions of both health authorities and community trusts. This means that for the first time all community health services come under the same umbrella. PCOs have a statutory responsibility to develop integrated primary care (and, in time, social care). In effect they are leading a new attempt to develop comprehensive primary health care.

There are major obstacles to achieving integrated primary health care, and the PCOs must overcome these. The obstacles include incompatible understandings of science, health and change, and until these are resolved different players will reluctantly co-exist rather than truly integrate.

Integrating a whole system of care requires whole-system learning which changes relationships between different people, both horizontally and vertically. This chapter discusses the meaning of learning, change and whole systems. The term 'whole system' is an idea, or mental model, that recognises the importance of connections between one thing and another. The question: 'What is the system of care for diabetes?' cannot be answered in any practical way unless an earlier question is resolved: 'What is the reason for asking?'

Localities for health could embody the ideas of whole-system learning and change, for example through 'practice-based commissioning' (a new policy in the UK to devolve the commissioning of services to local levels). A locality can be visualised as a 'cell' that enables internal interactivity and innovation, and through a 'semi-permeable membrane' makes carefully chosen external relationships to form networks for quality.

The contemporary political context, not just in the UK, seems favourable at present to allow experiments with the idea of whole-system learning and change. It will require all sectors to play a role. Educational institutions must teach systems thinking and the skills of shared leadership. Professional bodies must loudly proclaim the importance of whole-person care and multi-disciplinary working.

A worldwide need for integrated primary health care

In Chapter 9 I describe an international need for integrated primary health care. One main obstacle to achieving this identified by the WHO is the difficulty in integrating medical care with all other contributions to health and care. The difficulty of this connection has resulted in fragmented health care systems the world over.

It seems that horizontal multi-disciplinary team-working is just too difficult to achieve. But its importance is not disputed.

- In 1998 the Committee on the Quality of Health Care in America developed a strategy to improve the quality of health care. In 2001 it concluded that the American health care system was unable to adequately translate knowledge into quality practice because of fragmentation of effort, inadequate information systems and inability of individual effort to improve the quality of the system as a whole. It advocated the redesign of health services towards team-working, using insights from the science of complex adaptive systems.[1]
- WHO conferences in the 1990s resulted in the Ljubjana Charter. All European countries adopted this in 1996. It includes the principles of a broad vision for health, team-working, participation and fairness.
- In 2004 Berwick analysed the key lesson from developing nations about how to improve health care. He concluded: 'the full use of teams'.[2]

The UK is well positioned to achieve integrated primary health care that sustains. It has achieved a shift of resources to support it. It has achieved organisational infrastructure to lead it. Its politicians are describing an intention to achieve it.

Primary care trusts (PCTs) came into being in 2003 in England. In other parts of the UK they are called 'primary care organisations' (PCOs). They are large and network-like institutions which have absorbed many of the roles of both health authorities and community trusts. Each PCT/PCO serves a population of about 200 000 people. They hold the general practice contracts and the public health function. Soon they will also take responsibility for social care. PCT/PCOs have a statutory responsibility to integrate services. In effect they are charged to move towards the WHO idea of comprehensive primary health care (Chapter 9).

This means that, for the first time, all state provision for community services for health and social care will come under the same umbrella. Furthermore, this umbrella has a statutory responsibility to create integrated health and social care. It is intended to devolve commissioning for services to locality level (about 50 000 people). This is the size we found useful in Liverpool to facilitate local collaboration for multi-organisation innovations. It is small enough for practitioners and managers to develop good relationships and large enough to encourage healthy competition.

If the grand Alma Ata idea of comprehensive primary health care can be achieved anywhere, surely the UK can do it.

In the first part of this chapter I highlight some of the obstacles to achieving integrated primary health care and the potential of PCO localities to overcome these. I follow this with a tour of theories of learning and complex systems to show where lie the bodies of knowledge to conceptualise complex integration. I then explore what organisations and disciplines could take a lead for this.

Obstacles to achieving integrated primary health care

The WHO found huge obstacles to achieving integration when it tried, and failed, to operationalise the idea of comprehensive primary health care after the Alma Ata conference of 1978 (Chapter 9). Power, mismatch between needs and wants, and inadequate theory of organisations and systems are not the only problems. Different understandings of science, health and change mean that people aim for different things, use the same words to mean different things, and say things they do not mean. People may know in their hearts that what they say and do are not adequate reflections of what they mean, but they often do not have the language, the opportunity or even the courage, to examine this.

It will fall to those leading development and commissioning for whole geographic areas to grapple with the problems of these incompatible under-standings. I explore them in Part III.

In Chapter 9 I describe primary health care as a way of thinking about health for which all citizens and aspects of society have a responsibility. In Chapter 12 I argue that it helps to consider health to be the foundation for developing meaningful stories. Those who work to improve physical, social, mental and spiritual health are each working towards this broad goal. Integrated primary health care requires that state provision for health and social care is comple-mented with healthy public policy and social cohesion, facilitating the development of communities, organisations and systems, as well as individuals.

In Chapter 10 I describe general medical practice as a role particularly able to support vertical and horizontal integration of efforts for health and social care. However, our strong identification with scientific evidence to support our actions makes us less familiar with non-linear processes involved in organisational and systemic change. In Chapter 11 I propose three theories of knowledge that together may resolve this problem.

In Chapter 13 I argue that it is unhelpful to view whole-system change either as one 'big bang' transformation or as the steady march of a disciplined army. Instead, it can be seen as an ongoing dance of connected groups, each producing 'incremental revolutions'. An infrastructure of facilitation and communication helps these 'revolutions' to coalesce, or to enhance each other in other ways – and consequently integrate whole systems.

Crucial to achieving this complex synchrony of effort will be the development of local communities that are skilled at collaboration. In the UK the NHS policy of 'practice-based commissioning' could provide the structural opportunity for this. This policy is intended to bring clusters of general practices and other health workers together to develop services. This could result in localities becoming a prime focus for health care innovation. It could result in the following.

- Local integration of services: horizontally, through multi-disciplinary team-working, and vertically, through care pathways. Those who are skilled at community development, including the voluntary sector, schools and churches, could have a role in shaping local policy for multi-disciplinary collaboration.
- Regular whole-system events that enable diverse stakeholders to revisit their shared vision and develop co-ordinated plans.
- Projects that promote win–win transactions, such as Timebank (which enables people to gain community credits), 'one-stop shops' (which signpost an array of services) and arts programmes (which encourage creative interaction).
- Centres that support the development of shared leadership. Here, different disciplines can learn from and with each other, plan integrated services, develop shared-care records and amalgamate local information.
- Networks, and networks of networks, which cross organisational boundaries and broker coalitions of interest for quality.
- R&D systems[3] which help research and audit projects to operate hand-in-hand, and in response to local need. Established models that connect enquiry and action can be used, such as whole-system participatory action research[4,5] and action learning,[6] supported by academic or practitioner partnerships. Data from GP computer systems and other sources are amalgamated and fed back to stakeholders so they can learn.
- A cross-sectoral consortium of agencies that supports integration of efforts for quality, including research, audit, organisational development and leadership.
- Participation of trainee health workers of different disciplines. They can revisit the same locality year after year where they become temporary members of teams enquiring into local issues. In this way they will experience a broad understanding of health and see how things change year after year. Their personal projects will document their own development and the development of their case study. Each identifiable unit, for example a general practice, health visitors, pharmacists, social workers, can provide leaders for audit, research and organisational development. Together they can be supported to develop shared leadership for the locality. They could undertake university-accredited courses that help them to apply the theory of whole-system learning and change to their specific context, and at increasing levels of complexity.

What is whole-system learning and change?

Pause

What do you mean by the terms 'learning', 'whole-system' and 'change'?

Knowles,[7] makes this distinction between education and learning:

- Education is an activity undertaken or initiated by one or more agents that is designed to effect changes in the knowledge, skill and

attitudes of individuals, groups or communities. The term emphasises the educator, the agent of change who presents stimuli, and
reinforcement for learning and designs activities to induce change.
(p. 11)

- The term 'learning', by contrast, emphasizes the person in whom
the change occurs or is expected to occur. Learning is the act or
process by which behavioural change, knowledge, skills and attitudes are acquired. (p. 11)

Over the following six pages of his book, Knowles[7] analyses different interpretations of learning. Learning is:

- the mastery of what is already known, the extension or clarification
of meaning of one's experience, an organized, intentional process of
testing ideas relevant to problems (p.11)
- concerned with the acquisition of habits, knowledge and attitudes.
It enables the individual to make both personal and social adjustments (p.12)
- reflected in a change in behavior as a result of experience (p. 12)
- a process by which behavior is changed, shaped or controlled (p. 13)
- self actualisation (p. 15)
- a way to be in the world (p.15)
- five domains including motor skills, verbal information, intellectual
skills, cognitive strategies, attitudes (p. 16)
- six types of connections – cathexis, equivalence beliefs, field
experiences, field cognition modes, drive discriminations, and
motor patterns (p. 16)
- in three domains – cognitive, affective and psychomotor. (p. 16)

Knowles[7] concludes: 'It is certainly clear by now that learning is an elusive
phenomenon' (p. 16). And then:

> Key components of learning theorists' definition of learning serve as
> the foundation for our discussion of the definition of learning. These
> include: filling a need; learning as product; learning as process;
> learning as function; natural growth; control; shaping; development
> of competencies; fulfilment of potential; personal involvement; self-
> initiated; learner-evaluated; independent learning; and learning
> domains. (p. 17)

Knowles' analysis reminds us that learning and change are related. People and
organisations stagnate without ongoing changes that enrich them and help them
to fulfil their potential. Also, change is unavoidable. Everything is changing
around you and if you do not adapt to everything else you will be left out.
Learning and change are necessary aspects of a healthy society.

Organisational learning

In this book I draw particularly on the theories of organisational learning put
forward by Argyris and Schon because they make a connection between the
learning of an individual and the learning of groups, organisations and systems.

In the words of Swanwick, they help 'shift the focus to how the mind develops within its cultural setting'.[8] Learning is not the property solely of one person, but a 'socio-cultural progression from "newcomer" to "old-timer" '.[8] Organisations, communities and systems can learn, as well as individuals.

The relevance of the principles of organisational learning to quality general practice have long been recognised. Some primary care educationalists have systematically applied this understanding across whole areas.[9]

Argyris and Schon define three different types of learning: single-loop, double-loop and deutero-learning (see Chapter 2). They relate these to learning within whole organisations (Chapter 13).

The set of skills to lead change within a learning organisation have been described by Senge as five disciplines:[8]

- Systems thinking – recognising that everything is 'bound by invisible fabrics of interrelated systems'.
- Personal mastery – 'continually deepening and clarifying our personal vision, of focusing our energies, of developing patience, and of seeing reality objectively.
- Mental models – 'learning to unearth our personal pictures of the world, to bring them to the surface and hold them rigorously to scrutiny'.
- Building shared vision – 'holding a shared picture of the future we seek to create'.
- Team learning – 'allowing the group to discover insights not attainable individually . . . and recognising the patterns of interactions in teams that undermine learning'.

I consider that 'rigorous enquiry' is a sixth discipline – organisational learning requires that members are able to pose good questions and then answer them in reliable ways.

Systems theories

Central to the idea of a learning organisation is working with whole systems. This brings into view the management literature about whole systems.

The Open University course T306 describes 23 different influences on the five different branches of 'general system theory', 'systems approaches', 'first-' and 'second-order cybernetics', and 'information theory'.

Maturana and Varela[10] have influenced the development of second-order cybernetics. They write: 'the world everyone sees is not *the* world, but *a* world, which we bring forth with others' (p. 47).

Maturana[11] coins the idea of 'autopoiesis', literally 'self-creating' (p. 141). Here, he signals social constructionism, which maintains that: 'all socially significant dimensions of interaction . . . originate and are constructed in joint action'[12] (p. 179), and 'constructivism'[13]: what you see depends on the way you look. I describe these notions in Chapter 11.

Checkland describes hard and soft systems.[14] A 'hard system' is a linear idea – like the cardiovascular system, in which blood is pumped by the heart around the body in one direction. A care pathway is an example of a hard system. By contrast, a 'soft system' describes the multiple dynamic exchanges witnessed when multiple chemicals cross the membrane of a heart muscle cell. Team-working within a learning community is an example of a soft system.

Von Bertallanfy influenced general systems theory. He takes the idea of 'what-you-see-depends-on-how-you-look' idea into multiple interconnected systems:

> a system can be composed of smaller systems and can be part of a larger system . . . Consequently, the same organized entity can be regarded as either a system or a subsystem, depending on the observer's focus of interest.[15]

He described open systems: 'continually interacting with its environment. Open systems, as opposed to closed systems, sustain themselves by continually exchanging materials.'[15]

Capra describes a similar idea as a 'cell' – the 'basic form of life'.[10] A cell has a semi-permeable membrane that permits levels of complex internal interactions and adaptations and innovation that are not possible in a large soup of disorganised units. The membrane permits different things to cross selectively, allowing meaningful interaction with the external world.

These theorists are putting forward an image of a whole system which includes hard visible structures and complex dynamic adaptations. You can see both of these depending on which lens you use to look at the whole. You can switch lenses as much as you want.

Let me extend Capra's image a bit to apply it to a network of localities across many PCOs. First, look at one cell in your own hand. Witness the extraordinary complexity of interactions within this microscopic world. That cell connects in a meaningful way with multiple other cells to form a finger, a hand, a body, a whole person. Less visibly – but equally vitally – that whole person inter-connects with families, communities, towns and countries. At each place there are webs of relationships that maintain the integrity of the whole identity. If you want to see a cell there are plenty to see. If you want to see arms, families, countries – they are there too, all bound up in each other's ongoing co-creation. They are all engaged in a never-ending, complex dance of whole-system learning and change.

A locality is a cell within many other cells. Within the locality are many other cells that are in ongoing interaction with one another.

This is a 'hard systems' image: cell–finger–arms are connected in vertical hierarchical ways. Look deeper and you will see the horizontal 'soft system' idea of complex integration between skin and blood and bone, held together not by linear control but by mutual inter-dependence.

Here is the dynamic iterative interaction and exploration of possibilities within a cell. These movements are too many and too subtle to be predicted at a distance.

These theories can frame a theory of integrated primary health care which achieves both tangible visibility and dynamic interactivity. Each health care unit – small enterprises, networking institutions and localities – enables complex internal interactivity, learning and innovation. Externally, through its 'semi-permeable membrane' it develops multiple connections with other cells.

Applying systems ideas to UK primary health care

The King's Fund devised a series of models to facilitate whole-system learning and change in primary health care (Chapter 4).[16] Their account of their work defines a system as 'the people and organisations that connect around a shared purpose'.[16]

Diabetes care demonstrates the idea of a whole system. Involved are generalist and specialist medical practitioners, nurses, opticians, pharmacists, voluntary groups, social workers, housing, next-door neighbours. Each stakeholder can demonstrate simple, linear, direct relationships with others, such as a GP referring a patient to a renal specialist. But, even for simple monitoring of diabetes, the overall picture is of multiple relationships and cross-connections which evolve and change over time. In reality it is even more complicated than that. The system of care for people with diabetes overlaps with laboratory, ambulance and hospital admission systems. The system of care for insulin-dependent and non-insulin-dependent diabetes is different. The system for those with diabetes who are housebound, and those who are mobile, is different.

Of course, it goes further than that. All systems for diabetes care overlap with systems of care for other conditions – cardiovascular, eye and renal care. Each stakeholder will connect with multiple other systems that have nothing to do with diabetes at all. Very quickly, the idea of a whole system starts to look like an unmanageable mass of networks that are more likely to trip people up than help them. A whole system is best seen not as a static, all-inclusive megastructure, but as an idea that helps bring into view the different things that are relevant to deal with a concern.

A whole system is a mental model

The term 'whole system' is an idea, or mental model, that recognises the connections between one thing and another. The question: 'What is the system of care for diabetes?' cannot be answered in any meaningful way unless an earlier question is asked: 'What is the reason for asking?' If the reason is for a patient to access information, the system of concern is different from that when a doctor wants to know how to manage poor control in someone with diabetes.

Localities and 'nodes' make whole-system operating visible

For practical purposes, a whole system as a mental model is not enough. People often need to know where to go and what to do. This is the power of a locality. It is visible. It exists on a map. The people have names and faces. The rather theoretical language of mental models, virtual organisations and networks can find concrete grounding. Locality growth can be evaluated in very traditional ways – waiting times, cure rates, satisfaction scores, crime and school attendance rates.

To connect multiple localities 'nodes' are needed. A node is a junction where different paths cross. They are the places where different networks interconnect. Leaders work out where to put these, and guard them as places where different people can exchange ideas across boundaries. Nodes can be databases, coffee rooms, team meetings, learning centres and whole-system events. They are effective when they are learning spaces – places where participants explore what it is like for others, learn how to do things differently, and consider how to change things in harmony. Events at nodes need to be advertised well in advance and the people who need to be there must be able to get there. You cannot anticipate what will come out of them, because this emerges from the creative interactions within them. Nodes generate potential for change. In Chapter 6 I describe how to plan where to put nodes.

Whole-system events

The King's Fund techniques and other whole-system events (Chapter 15) can facilitate whole-system learning and change within localities. Whole-system events enable large numbers of different people to develop shared purpose and devise a co-ordinated multi-faceted, multi-agency plan.

At whole-system events consensus emerges about shared vision and a set of projects to move towards this. Teams are set up to lead them. Their progress is reviewed at a series of future meetings where the stakeholders make explicit the new status quo and rethink the next steps. This allows periods where people from the whole system stand back and look at things, learn from and with each other how the system is working, and what future possibilities are coming into view. It also allows periods when people go away with a mandate to work on their detailed plans. This allows the old organisational development idea of 'freeze–unfreeze' to be set inside a much more dynamic process of whole-system inter-activity, allowing the conclusions of multiple discrete projects to converge at the same time, and be considered as a whole.

A large number of seemingly isolated projects can happen at the same time. But, because they were devised and revised from a shared vision, they have greater potential to coalesce or otherwise integrate with each other at a later stage. The faster things change the closer together need to be the times to stand back. On the other hand, holding meetings closer together gives less time for participants to act on the learning of the previous stage – a balance needs to be struck. Different situations require different meeting intervals. Leaders can speed up or slow down change by altering these intervals.

The process of inter-disciplinary learning at whole-system events can quickly reveal systemic problems. For example, it is common for different systems to record the immunisation of children without any communication between them. Ongoing cycles of freeze–unfreeze, coupled with ongoing discussions between the various teams, allow these systems to adapt to the others in a managed way, and, over time, transform into a new interconnected whole. How to plan this is explored in Chapter 6.

Where should we look for leadership for whole-system learning and change?

Pause

Which organisations and disciplines do you think should lead integrated primary health care?

Which disciplines and organisations provide the natural source of leadership for whole-system learning and change? Visionary individuals and serendipity are not enough. Certainly different PCOs will make things work in ways that depend on who is interested and able. But planning is also needed.

In the UK, PCO boards and professional executive committees are intended to provide leadership. They can facilitate team-working vertically, though care pathways and intermediate care, and horizontally, through locality commissioning and trans-disciplinary projects. They can help practitioners and patients to navigate the whole system by skilful commissioning of computer decision support, maps of care pathways and educational courses which promote reflective practice, collaborative enquiry and systems thinking. Even if there is future restructuring there will remain a need for this role of shared leadership for integrated care throughout whole geographic areas.

But the practice and theory to make it all work is quite different from the formative training of the individuals expected to step into these roles. For example, medical students learn little about team-working, trainee GPs are expected to consider audit solely as the measuring of quantitative standards and even established GPs have no training in systems thinking. Which disciplines should society prepare for a more sophisticated understanding of learning, change and enquiry within whole systems?

The question is important because educationalists need to know how to revise plans for formative and ongoing education; professional bodies need to consider the practical implications of expanded roles; and health care managers need to provide opportunities for people to step into them. But who should they be?

A thin answer is that truly integrated primary health care requires all citizens to be skilled at whole-system working. This is unrealistic in the short term, but could be a long-term vision. People described by the Urban Partnerships Group as 'boundroids' are likely candidates (http://homepages.phonecoop.coop/julian.pratt/index.htm). These are people who have feet in different camps and do not fit neatly into any one 'box'. Boundroid GPs include sessional doctors, GPs with special interest, and others with portfolio careers. Such practitioners habitually work in different parts of the system and consequently have windows into different worlds of experience and knowledge. From these windows they can better see cross-system opportunities, and facilitate bridges to support integrated efforts for health. The potential of boundroids to facilitate cross-organisational boundaries could be developed systematically. Presently they are often marginalised – naturally, because they operate at the margins.

Another answer is that it should fall within the remit of those with a vocation for caring for the whole person, because they will better understand the importance of human relations. In this case nursing is a likely discipline – after all most facilitators of change in the past 15 years have been nurses. Another possible answer is those who have a good understanding of power – it should be noted that occupational health projects supported by the Trades Council have worked successfully facilitated collaboration between general practice and trade unionists in many UK cities. But there are many other candidates – social workers, lay health workers, mental health workers and the voluntary sector.

GPs and public health practitioners have a particular reason to find the role of whole-system facilitator appealing. They both already have multiple windows into aspects of life through regular contact with large numbers of other disciplines. They already orchestrate complex inter-communication between many different people – public health through the 'new public health'[17] (Chapter 9) and GPs through whole-person care (Chapter 10). It would be coherent to the origins of both to become formally trained in whole-system theory and practice.

One conclusion is that multi-disciplinary teams are needed for this role of shared leadership. We successfully developed this model in Liverpool in 1993. Four multidisciplinary teams of local practitioners were trained to lead locality reflection and action.[18,19]

A home for leaders of integrated primary health care

Applied academic centres are needed to support the development of shared leadership. To ensure ongoing development of sequential cohorts of leaders these centres need to have good partnerships with PCOs. They will also need to connect with similar centres, nationally and internationally, to provide a global network with multiple opportunities for developing advanced skills of leadership for integrated primary health care.

At these centres participants can learn from and with each other, as well as learning the theory and skills of whole-system learning and change. They can use their real-life work as their personal case studies, which contribute to their credits of academic achievement. This would have the effect of in-service training to support the development of practical things, such as integrated protocols, integrated databases and integrated evaluation, as well as their personal leadership skills. The students from one year can be the supervisors of subsequent cohorts, creating a 'spiral curriculum', where the same theory is visited at increasing levels of complexity.

Strategic health authorities

Strategic health authorities (SHAs) relate to several PCOs within a sector. The role of the SHA is to ensure quality services and collaborative working across the area. For this reason they are particularly concerned with developing leadership that spans the PCOs.

Networks

A network is a 'virtual organisation' which crosses organisational boundaries and consequently can facilitate collaborative working. In England, teaching PCTs, primary care research networks and clinical networks are examples of networks with a responsibility to facilitate collaborative practice between PCOs.

PCOs, professional bodies and higher education institutions need to work in partnership

PCOs, professional bodies and higher education institutions could provide organisational support for an infrastructure of whole-system leadership.

Historically, PCOs have created communication systems and supported teamworking, so this would make relevant to present times an old role. It will fall to the professional bodies to argue how the values of comprehensive whole-person care can be developed in the new National Health Service (NHS) structures. In the past such groups have taken a visionary role, so this, too, would make an old role relevant to present times.

It will fall to higher education institutions to claim the role of teaching leadership for integrated primary health care. Many universities already have considerable experience of this, and have been developing relationships with their local PCOs and particularly with 'teaching PCTs', which have a remit to support learning across several PCTs.

The NHS Institute for Innovation and Improvement (www.institute.nhs.uk) has a role to support service transformation, technology and product innovation, leadership development and learning.

Interdependence of individuals and communities

In the UK, a Labour government was elected in 1997, after a decade of seemingly unstoppable individualism and free market philosophy under a Conservative administration. This made it acceptable to talk about creative tensions between different needs.

Both 'top-down' and 'bottom-up' approaches to change were advocated within a structured framework for development. The language of 'rights and responsibilities' emerged, signalling a need for balance between both. The language of 'partnership working', 'diversity management' and 'equity' gained prominence.

This shift in language signalled a change from the idea that change comes from choosing *either* one *or* another approach, to the idea that *both* one *and* other approaches can be complementary. The term that was most used to summarise this more complex idea was 'The Third Way'. In his book of this title, Giddens described how the psychology of the individual and the sociology of communities are equally important.[20] However, Giddens did not offer a theory of how these different understandings can be integrated.

In Part III I offer such a theory. Individual identity and social culture are not so much given as co-created through interaction in the world. This interaction forms webs of relationships and multiple inter-connected life stories. Each individual wants his or her story to be coherent in order to retain the integrity of their sense of self, so individuals are motivated to act when they see potential for this. Language cannot do justice to the complexity of this dynamic process. Subconscious motivations and non-verbal communications powerfully affect what happens.

This results in a complex relationship between individual and collective identities. There is no such thing as 'a community'. Instead, there are multiple overlapping and inter-dependent networks of relationships. I explain in Chapter 12 that each person seeks to describe him- or herself as the lead actor in the feature film that is their life story. Social relationships are part of that story. Neither individuals nor communities stand alone – they are related to each other as parts are related to wholes.

This suggests a need to reframe the ideas of individualism and socialism to be more interdependent – both are needed. However, each brings a different set of related ideas. Individualism promotes ideas of vertical 'ladder climbing', dominating hierarchical authority, and the linear notion of 'representation'. Socialism promotes ideas of horizontal community relationships, equitable consensus authority and the complexity notion of 'participation'.

The inter-dependence of the individual and the group suggests that neither the idea of individualism nor socialism on its own is meaningful. The political stances of 'left wing' and 'right wing' might be better reframed to describe different emphasis on participatory and representational processes. At different times for different reasons both are desirable, but the ideal balance in specific contexts needs to be debated.

References

1 Plsek P (2000) *Crossing the Quality Chasm – A New Health System for the 21st Century.* National Academy of Sciences, Washington DC.
2 Berwick DM (2004) Lessons from developing nations on improving health care. *BMJ.* **328**: 1124–9.
3 Ison R and Russell D (2000) *Agricultural Extension and Rural Development.* Cambridge University Press, Cambridge.
4 Thomas P, Oni L, Alli M, St Hilaire J, Smith A, Leavey C *et al.* (2005) Antenatal screening for haemoglobinopathies in primary care – a whole system participatory action research project. *British Journal of General Practice.* **55**: 424–8.
5 Thomas P, McDonnell J, McCulloch J, While A, Bosanquet N and Ferlie E (2005) Increasing capacity for innovation in large bureaucratic primary care organizations – a whole system participatory action research project. *Annals of Family Medicine* **3**: 312–17.
6 Revans R (1998) *ABC of Action Learning.* Lemos & Crane, London.
7 Knowles M (1998) *The Adult Learner.* Butterworth-Heinemann, Woburn, MA.
8 Swanwick T (2005) Informal learning in postgraduate medical education: from cognitivism to 'culturism'. *Medical Education.* **39**: 859–64.
9 Downey P and Waters M (2005) Developing the primary health care team as a learning organisation: a new model using problem-based learning. *Education for Primary Care.* **16**: 301–7.
10 Capra F (2003) *The Hidden Connections.* Flamingo, St Ives.
11 Carr A (2000) Theories that focus on belief systems. In: A Carr (ed) *Family Therapy. Concepts, Processes and Practice.* John Wiley, London.
12 Shotter J (2000) *Conversational Realities – Constructing Life through Language.* Sage, London.
13 Guba E (1990) *The Paradigm Dialog.* Sage, Newbury Park, CA.
14 Checkland P (1995) *Systems Thinking, Systems Practice.* Wiley, Bath.
15 Nichols M and Schwartz R (1998) The fundamental concepts of family therapy. In: M Nichols and R Schwartz (eds) *Family Therapy, Concepts and Methods* (4e). Allyn and Bacon, London.
16 Pratt J, Gordon P and Plamping D (1999) *Working Whole Systems: Putting Theory into Practice in Organisations.* King's Fund, London.
17 Ashton J and Seamore H (1988) *The New Public Health.* Open University Press, Buckingham.
18 Graver LD, Springett J, Sands R and Reason P (1997) *Evaluation of the Local Multidisciplinary Facilitation Teams.* John Moores University Centre for Health Studies, Liverpool.
19 Thomas P and Graver LD (1997) The Liverpool intervention to promote teamwork in general practice: an action research approach. In: P Pearson and J Spencer (eds) *Promoting Teamwork in Primary Care – A Research Based Approach.* Arnold, London.
20 Giddens A (1998) *The Third Way.* Polity Press, Malden.

Part II

Developing your leadership skills

This second part of the book is intended to develop your skills of leading within complex situations. You will find it most useful if you bring your own real-life situation as a case study to use when going through the material. I suggest you keep your own notes to record what you have learned, and what you would like to learn from other resources, or on other days. Writing things down helps to articulate and reinforce learning. There are different paths for you to choose through these five chapters, as follows.

- You can get an overall feel of the areas covered by first reading the summaries, the images and models, or the examples.
- You can use the 'Things you can do to . . .' to focus on specific aspects. Each chapter has four of these and they are intended to prepare for a half-day workshop within a leadership course.
- You can do the exercises at the end of each chapter to relate the ideas directly to your needs.
- You can work through the example scenarios – these will be most helpful if they resemble your own situation.

Three scenarios run through all five chapters:

- the development of a general practice
- the development of a community hospital
- locality health care development.

The scenarios reflect three different kinds of organisation which have different ways of exercising authority and mechanisms to facilitate innovation:

- a small enterprise, which comprises a multi-disciplinary team with shared vision and plans
- a large institution, which houses multiple semi-independent programmes of work
- a network where members dip in and out of many activities, depending on their interest at the time.

At the start of each chapter I pose a new twist to the stories and invite you to describe how you would deal with this. At the end of the chapter I ask you whether the chapter has helped you to think differently about your plan, and what you have learnt.

These different kinds of organisation exercise authority and facilitate innovation in different ways.

General practice: a small enterprise

A general practice is an example of a 'small enterprise'. Here, a small number of people provide a gateway to other parts of the health service. They treat and refer patients with every kind of illness. It is possible for team members to know each other and what each other does. To be effective in its daily business the enterprise gives tasks to individuals who have the appropriate skills to perform them. Power is usually formally held by a small number of named 'partners', who manage the organisation. 'Corridor conferences' often result in spur of the moment policy, which can lead to fast innovation. However, this can also exclude whoever was not in the corridor at that time. Commonly, there is an 'oral tradition' in that the 'rules' are not written down. Instead the partners provide the organisational memory and interpret organisational 'rules'. In small enterprises there are large numbers of formal and informal ways for team members to influence direction because of the everyday interaction between different disciplines. Innovation commonly happens from the enthusiasm of a few team members – often going ahead with little reference to what has happened in other places.

A community hospital: an institution

A community hospital is an example of an 'institution'. Institutions are large organisations which relate closely to other organisations that are established features of an area. Despite often dominating the imagination of funders and the public alike (not to mention the landscape), they tend to stifle innovation. Institutions can be, well, institutionalised (*Chambers 21st Century Dictionary*: 'dull, regimented and impersonal; e.g. a long-stay hospital or prison'). This is because they host a range of different programmes of work in which large numbers of people have little opportunity to be creative together. To be effective in its daily business the institution delegates authority to individual managers, who oversee others to perform service tasks. Power is held within a bureaucratic structure. Directors oversee extensive portfolios of work. Accountability is to line managers, who make judgements according to the rules of the organisation. The rules are multiple, written down and challenged politically. Organisational learning and change is usually slow, and commonly happens through political champions and within named units. Trans-disciplinary learning and external collaboration can help innovation in these bureaucracies.[1] This recognition has led to increased interest in the idea of a 'network organisation'.[2]

A geographic locality: a network

A primary care locality is an example of a 'network'. Networks are virtual organisations that connect people who share an interest. They are effective at innovation by facilitating coalitions of interest. Different members with have different specific interests and will want to dip in and out of things when they want to. In a network no one has formal power over other members – only the power of persuasion, peer pressure and contracts for specific work. Members have no formal accountability to the network as a whole – only to the commitments they make to undertake projects and to take network roles.

Small enterprises, institutions and networks use different ways to learn and change because of their different sizes and diversity of stakeholders and through using different kinds of power. However, each approach also has weaknesses as well as strengths and they can each benefit by adopting features of the others. A small enterprise needs some rules, as in an institution, to stop powerful people from changing plans in an ad hoc way and excluding other team members. An institution needs informal and formal inter-departmental networking if it is to counter the stifling effect of its bureaucratic structures. A network needs strong institutions to protect it.

References

1 Thomas P, McDonnell J, McCulloch J, While A, Bosanquet N and Ferlie E (2005) Increasing capacity for innovation in large bureaucratic primary care organizations – a whole system participatory action research project. *Annals of Family Medicine*. **3**: 312–17.
2 Hatch MJ (1997) *Organization Theory – Modern, Symbolic, and Postmodern Perspectives*. Oxford University Press, Oxford.

Chapter 4

Moving the story forward

Summary

The terms 'leader', 'manager' and 'facilitator' were born out of a time when change was considered to be a simple and linear process. These concepts need to be reinterpreted in the light of modern-day understandings that change involves complex adaptation of different factors that may at first sight seem unrelated.

Change in complex situations can be seen as play, and leadership as story-weaving.

Leadership for integration is advanced team-working. An infrastructure of facilitation and communication could develop networks of high performing teams.

Leaders recognise that all things are connected in webs of relationships, and you will need disciplined techniques to quickly appraise where are the best places to apply effort. Different kinds of insights can reveal usefully different things about situations.

Leaders develop networks and teams to facilitate ongoing learning and change. Crucial to this are 'learning spaces' – safe environments where people learn from, and with, each other, and can explore uncomfortable things. Theory and techniques that help this come from adult learning principles, large-group interventions and teambuilding. Leaders connect learning spaces, creating networks of networks that facilitate 'whole-system conversations'.

Leaders help people to see both woods and trees. They see how whole forests are growing, and the relevance of small saplings within them. Leadership helps people from all parts of the forest to contribute to its healthy development.

Leaders help people to contribute by first involving them in conversations about an issue, asking what is the relevance of their work, or their life as a whole, to the issue? What are the needs of the services in connection with it? What would they actually like to do about it? Leaders then keep those people in conversations as things unfold, seizing opportunities to motivate for learning and action.

Take the example of diabetes care. From conferences, research/audit or personal experience come multiple observations about which parts of the system work, and which do not. Multi-disciplinary workshops generate specific ideas about what to do with these glitches. This may result in new communication systems between professionals, patient information leaflets about self-management and even new ways to treat diabetes itself.

Testing out these ideas generates knowledge which can be fed back into other conversations at a later stage. Predictable times for feedback help people to anticipate when they can contribute to later discussions.

The result is a community of practitioners and managers who care about good diabetes care, and who are aware that change in one part of the system may cause problems in other parts. Participants become rehearsed at moving between the parts and the wholes, and in devising projects that solve short-term problems in ways that build long-term infrastructure for learning and change.

Leaders constantly shift their gaze between focused detail and the bigger picture. They set up cycles of enquiry in projects that keep the right people thinking together and in touch with each other's thoughts. This form of leadership may not look like leadership at all, at least not in a traditional sense of 'leaders and followers'. This role helps individuals and teams to see the relevance of their immediate work to broader systems to which they are connected. It helps them to form relationships with others with whom they can develop innovative ideas.

In Chapter 1 I explained that when considering processes of integration it is not helpful to distinguish between leaders, managers and facilitators. Each is concerned with moving things forward in complex situations. In the terms of this book, leadership is also a team activity in which everyone can be a hero at appropriate times. Leaders can be the quiet ones who support others to take responsibilities and give people space to test out their ideas. Leaders map systems of concern and explain this map to others. This helps people to navigate the system under their own steam, in the same way that railway maps and timetables help people to make complicated journeys. Leaders aim not to pull more and more tasks onto themselves, but to build a sustainable infrastructure of facilitation and communication to enable ongoing adaptation to each other's progress.

This description of leaders represents a marked departure from the traditional idea of 'heroic leaders'. The heroic plate-spinner leaves onlookers in awe at the skill and daring needed to keep so many plates spinning. There will still be a need for brave and talented heroes, prepared to take such risks. But more commonly leaders will find out where the plates are, and get to know the spinners. They will encourage them to try new ways of spinning, and offer them ways to learn from and with other plate spinners. This style of leader still makes 'tough' decisions – sacking people, for example. But they get to such moments of crisis less often because they will have spotted problems at an early stage, and provided support and ongoing review to resolve them.

This image of leadership is advanced team-working. Leaders recognise that the task is more than any one person can deal with, and that different team members appeal to different constituencies. They naturally develop a network of high-performing teams which span the organisations and disciplines concerned, gaining a rich understanding of the whole story. In this chapter I suggest that leadership is a function that moves forwards whole stories in complex situations.

Choose your case study: facilitating a shared understanding of the story

An introduction to this section can be found at the start of Part II.

Developing a general practice

You are leading change in a general practice to increase its performance in the new GP contract. The practice has 8000 patients, in a deprived urban area. English is a second language for many of your patients and about three consultations each day are held through an interpreter. There are three full-time doctors, who are practice partners. There are four GP assistants, who do varying numbers of clinical sessions, together equalling approximately one whole-time equivalent. You have one practice nurse, a registrar (a qualified doctor in GP training) and a counsellor who does two half-day sessions a week. There are 12 receptionists/administrators and they work hours that suit their other commitments.

Your challenge is to increase an array of targets, including the number of patients who have had their blood pressure recorded, smokers counselled and children who have had full immunisations. You also want to move forwards a project that interests you. You know that this will require a level of data recording and cross-disciplinary communication which is new to everyone. Traditionally there have been few formal meetings and they rarely reach conclusions that are followed through. Practitioners input information into the computer in different ways. There is a fast throughput of reception staff and some do not feel appreciated. Nobody seems to know who is a part of their extended team.

Write down how you would get everyone to have a better understanding of the whole story.

Developing a community hospital

You are leading change in a community hospital to make it more integrated with primary care activities. It has so far been largely focused on secondary care. The hospital has 30 beds in two wards, which consultants from a large teaching hospital use whenever the teaching hospital is full. The consultants also use the beds for rehabilitation and as surgical beds for day-case general surgery. Several hospital consultants hold outpatient clinics there. Minor surgery and phlebotomy are undertaken in a small emergency unit. The community hospital is the base for community nurses and health visitors, and houses a set of community services, including podiatry, physiotherapy and dietetics. However, these operate as stand-alone services and their practitioners have had little impact on the plans.

Your challenge is to facilitate a plan agreed by all involved and, in particular, to achieve a more coherent and thoughtful primary care voice. So far the main need expressed by GPs has been GP-accessed beds for respite care. A good financial case had been made for other proposals: a medical insurance company wants to develop a ward for private patients; hospital surgeons want overnight beds for patients to permit more major surgery to be undertaken; geriatricians want to site a day care centre there. The proposals are far more than the hospital can deal with. Many people are angry, suspicious and frustrated.

Write down how you would get everyone to have a better understanding of the whole story.

Developing a primary care locality

You are leading change in a locality of 100 000 people to help integrate local services. Here, 20 general practices are at different stages of development: some are unable to undertake even simple computer searches, while others lead research and teach students. There is very little local communication. At the local hospital different primary care practitioners work in isolation: health visitors and district nurses; podiatry; physiotherapy; dietetics and counselling. A handful of consultants from the two secondary care hospitals see outpatients in the community hospital, including mental health, geriatrics, respiratory medicine (mainly TB screening) and (minor) general surgery.

Your challenge is to get everyone working together to increase locality communication and co-ordinated service development.

Write down how you would get everyone to have a better understanding of the whole story.

An image of leadership: Mary Poppins

Mary Poppins* was a leader in a complex situation. She was invited into a dysfunctional organisation and by getting its members to sing silly songs and jump into pictures she helped all of them to step out of their usual selves, review their roles and values, and create something new and better. She set the scene by clarifying what the job was, how people should behave towards each other and when their contract would end. Her intervention, as viewed by the movie watcher, allowed people to review their context, culture and appreciation of each other, and develop new relationships and shared projects through which they transformed their whole system – the whole system learned. This created a new organisational culture that was more effective, more coherent and more healthy.

Those who facilitate organisational change are familiar with Poppins' methods. Her scene-setting is aims and ground rules, silly songs are icebreakers, and jumping into pictures is role play. The facilitator helps the participants to map and then reflect on their whole context. Following principles of adult learning[1] and action science[2] the facilitator engages the participants in a systemic, collaborative enquiry,[3] using visioning,[4] games[5,6] and large-group interventions[7] to test out new ways of doing things.

Organisational learning

Poppins gives an image of change as play. She suggests that leadership is story-weaving – the various actors test out new roles and ways of relating to each other and rewrite their scripts. Leadership helps them to recognise both the good and

*The 1964 Walt Disney classic *Mary Poppins* included a surreal mix of cartoons and trick photography. By engaging an unhappy family in positive interaction through games and song, they developed new relationships and a new sense of their shared purpose.

the harm they cause through their habitual actions. They come to see what they can do practically to change things in synchrony. They become motivated to do it. They identify things inside themselves they don't like – and they change these. These inner transformations alter their external behaviour. Poppins helps people to value the things that they already have. She helps them to see what is solid to build from and what things are pulling the whole story backwards. She helps participants to find better words to express what they mean, and to believe in themselves. She helps people to see truths they are afraid to look at.

The temptation in stressful situations is to retreat into a defensive, combative or authoritarian style. Poppins showed how an open, engaging and equalising style is more effective – an appreciative and playful game makes it easier for people to work outside their comfort zones and take calculated risks. She shows the power of experiential learning – when you experience something you understand it in a way that is deeper than mere words. Experience helps something to become part of your hidden inner world – your whole identity – rather than merely the words you use to discuss ideas with others.

At the end of the game participants return to almost exactly where they were before they started, except with new eyes. They are better able to see everyday potential to which they had become blinded through overfamiliarity or through overindulgence with their own concerns. They become ready, willing and able to try out new ways of doing things. They come to these conclusions themselves and may not recognise her leadership role in bringing about their learning and change. Not everyone needs to be a Mary Poppins, but everyone needs to understand the process of systemic change, and to engage willingly.

Poppins used shared leadership

Mary Poppins did not do this alone. She had different teams, which understood why she was doing things the way she did. They, too, laughed and danced and reassured the more anxious that it was safe to stay involved without knowing exactly what was going to happen. Each had their turn of being in the spotlight. Each was a leader in their own right and appealed to different constituencies.

Poppins is the organisational development consultant who is paid to facilitate a project and leaves at the end of the contract. When the wind changed direction Poppins left, flying off to an unnamed place. In primary care the need is too great to rely on external consultants and to allow such talent to go elsewhere. We need to find ways to embed these skills within health care systems. We need to develop and look after these people, and build teams of leaders with them who will in time take similar roles. Health services can do this by helping leaders to 'move on' but remain geographically in the same place. Co-ordinated programmes can help practitioners and managers to move in and out of these roles.

Pause

What image do you have of yourself as a leader?

A model of leadership within complex situations

This model (Figure 4.1) shows things a leader works with, or puts in place, in complex situations, so that people can engage with each other creatively.

On the far left of the figure are 'individual life stories'. In the case of diabetes these could be patients, medical practitioners, specialist nurses and self-help groups. Each tradition carries different expectations, different language, and different kinds of power and knowledge. 'Social forces' influence them constantly.

The boxes represent 'whole-system events' or meetings. You are likely to initiate some, join or watch others, and ignore most. They enable conversations between people from different parts of the system. An annual stakeholder conference for diabetes care is an example, attracting those who are interested in diabetes.

'Pilot projects' test new ideas. They can be short or long term, central or lateral to the main storyline. Leaders are skilled at choosing projects that are 'do-able', build capacity, and are insightful about the challenges of the journey ahead.

Policy formalises progress made. It legitimises others to adopt the understandings that have emerged. It also helps resources to flow to support activity. Leaders are skilled at writing policy which facilitates ongoing reflection and action, as well as giving clear direction. This encourages new ideas to emerge at a later stage.

'Surprises' are unexpected events. They can be associated with the leaving or arrival of significant individuals, new government policy, a clash of ideologies, the ending or starting of funding. Leaders are skilled at turning these to advantage.

'Networks' are connections between people who share an interest. The more people put their hearts into a shared project the stronger will be these connections. Leaders are skilled at releasing the potential of networks to connect and integrate different efforts for health.

'Guiding vision' is the lodestone. It is where the compass points about the general direction of travel. Leaders are skilled at facilitating shared vision, and helping people to take steps towards it.[8]

Examples of change as play

Residential teambuilding workshops

The Health Education Authority model of residential teambuilding workshops allowed general practice teams to describe shared vision and to design health promotion clinics.[9] Four or more multi-disciplinary teams, each with four to ten members, lived together for three days. Each team developed a plan for heart disease prevention, and was introduced to group learning techniques such as games, ground rules and role-play. Structured interaction with other teams and timely presentations and exercises were used to broaden their thinking. This had the effect of improving whole-practice team-working, as well as producing a plan for heart disease prevention and management. Follow-up by a facilitator at six weeks and six months helped to prevent loss of momentum.

These events were organised by an inter-agency 'local organising team' with senior management support.[10] This group planned and facilitated the team-

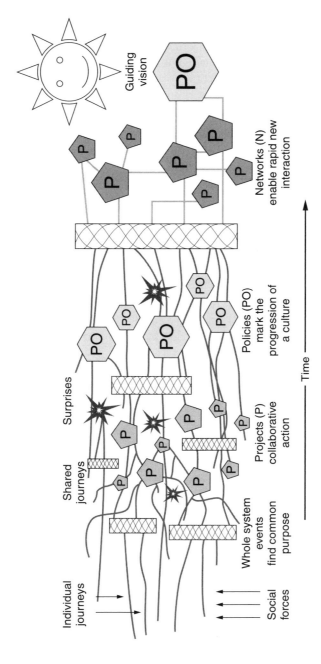

Figure 4.1 A model of leadership within complex situations.

building workshops. They also facilitated the development of cross-organisational collaborative projects, and policy which improved relationships throughout the whole system.

In Liverpool we adapted these workshops to support leadership development for multiple purposes, involving health visitors, practice nurses, GPs, district nurses, community psychiatric nurses, social workers, school nurses, health authority managers, practice managers, voluntary workers, trade unionists and lay health workers. Some teams went on to facilitate whole-system events and locality learning and change.

King's Fund whole-system interventions

Several models are described. One involved the Newcastle and North Tyneside Health Authority strengthening community-based services at the same time as closing hospital beds.[11] This developed closer relationships with the City Council, universities and voluntary groups:

> They brought everyone together in 1995. About 200 people attended the first event, 'milling around wondering what was going to happen'. Sitting around large round tables participants told their stories and expressed their concerns and hopes. Small-group–large-group iterations gathered a wealth of intelligence and next steps were agreed. One of the emerging themes was care of the elderly. This resulted in a 40-strong planning group that met over time to establish relationships and plan projects. In 1997 another whole-system event was facilitated using the technique called 'real time strategic change'.[12] This tested a draft strategy with a wide range of people and produced a new atmosphere of mutual understanding from which came initiatives such as a sheltered housing scheme shared between the housing department and a community health trust. (p. 81)

The Gladwell project [13]

> A team of facilitators from the consulting network Whole Systems Development provided support for self-governance of a neighbourhood. Through action learning groups and a sequence of large group meetings, they achieved widening circles of participation. This developed new leaders, allowing the original ones to move on to other things. (p. 40)

In these examples, people of diverse experience stepped out of their usual roles and played games together. They listened to the insights of people whose perspective they would normally not consider, developed networks between different institutions and devised multiple complementary projects that had a combined effect that was more than the sum of the parts. Patient and persistent follow-through resulted in highly performing multi-disciplinary teams able to work across boundaries and influence things at all levels of the health care system.

Things you can do to help the story evolve

Anticipate your future support needs

You have considerable power to secure the support you need for success when you enter a new situation. Gaining agreement at the outset of how you will approach the work will help to avoid later unhelpful interference and gain timely support.

The model of complex adaptation described above (Figure 4.1) leads you to expect everything to be connected in webs of relationships that the people 'inviting you in' may not recognise themselves – you must gain agreement from them to explore these and to share with them your assessment at an early stage.

The image of Mary Poppins leads you to see yourself as a facilitator of change in people's relationships as they weave their stories together. You may need promises of support to deal with any backlash from this process, which some will find confronting.

Those who invite you in must recognise that change involves different stages and they must take their part along the way. Even on the first day you may be able to see what timeline is needed to achieve what you want. Your employers must play their part when needed, acting quickly to seize an advantage or help you out of trouble. Raising expectations about these at the beginning may make them more prepared to act later on.

The chapters of Part II help to anticipate other things you will need.

- Helping people to enquire and learn together (Chapter 5).
- Building the infrastructure for ongoing learning and change (Chapter 6).
- Having the right information at the right time (Chapter 7).
- Looking after yourself (Chapter 8).

You can anticipate each of these at the outset.

There are things you need to promise yourself. These include using the project to develop your own self, including addressing your own weaknesses. You can highlight the potential of a proposed project to do this by drawing your life-line and considering what you need for your next steps (Chapter 14). Try sharing this analysis with someone you trust.

There are practical things you need to have in place:

- systems for recording and retrieving information and checking things have been done
- access to information, for example, libraries, websites and literature search facilities
- support for communication, for example administration, e-mail.

Implications for the clinical encounter

Each patient will have a set of future support needs – medical, social, financial – you can help them to see these.

Implications for running organisations and crafting policy

Organisations need to develop leaders who are capable of anticipating future problems and developing their own support systems to deal with them.

Implications for yourself

Anticipating your future needs for support will help you to move from one priority to another without losing your balance.

Appraise situations quickly

To get a good start in a new situation you need to understand it quickly. One technique that can help is 'rapid appraisal', which requires an understanding of the story so far from different perspectives. Rapid appraisal uses: written literature; personal observations; and interviews of key informants. Your appraisal should help you to make interpretations you had not considered at the outset, as well as allowing you to record your first impressions and gut instincts.

You need to map the situation to show how everything connects, and display the power relations. You can use an established genogram technique. The boundary you have agreed around the focus of your work may need to be revised to check that it is the best one to achieve what you want to achieve in the time you have.

Your rapid appraisal will help you to draw a picture similar to the model described above (Figure 4.1), replacing the generic labels with the real-life situation. It will:

- describe the various individual and shared stories and the social forces that shape them
- reveal who attends what meetings and what projects and policies are developed through them
- reveal various subgroups, alliances and networks that administer authority and power
- reveal what vision the stakeholders say they have and the extent to which their actions are true to that vision
- anticipate future surprises.

There are formal models that you can seek out and use. Rapid appraisal has been used by the WHO to assess community health needs[14] – participating researchers build an information pyramid that helps local people to see better their whole context. 'Rapid institutional appraisal' has been used by the Open University for staff induction – new staff members use semi-structured interviews and group work to understanding the whole university, surface issues of importance to their department and build relations.[15] 'Rapid reconnaissance' has been used within qualitative research to enter a research field quickly – members of interdisciplinary teams conduct informal interviews to produce an initial qualitative portrayal of the whole situation.[16]

Do not be put off by these impressive-sounding examples! A rapid appraisal can be devised without using an established framework. Your invitation to enter a situation will be accompanied by an initial analysis of the situation. Initial conversations, early gut feelings, observations and literature may point the way towards expanding this understanding. An exercise in mapping the system may reveal useful places to explore (Chapter 14). When interviewing people you can gain broad insights by asking general and specific questions about the past, and about the future. For example, questions about the past might be 'Tell me the history of the place?' (general) and 'Who have been the movers and shakers so far?' (specific). Questions about the future might be 'What is your vision for the future?' (general) and 'What are the obstacles to achieving this? Or, 'What would success look like?' (specific). Bringing together general and specific views about the past and the future, as perceived by different people, can reveal tensions and potentials which may be invisible at first sight.

Implications for the clinical encounter

You can ask patients general and specific questions about their past and future, to see more of the person beyond the diagnoses.

Implications for running organisations and crafting policy

Rapid appraisal can be used for the induction of new employees.

Implications for yourself

Rapid appraisal techniques will help you to get the measure of new situations quickly, in both your personal and professional lives.

Initiate whole-system conversations

Whether the whole system is two people or many organisations, ongoing conversations can:

- keep people connected
- clarify useful differences
- result in practical new ways of doing things.

Whole-system conversations are more than talk. They help people to puzzle together, think, reflect and produce new ideas. Leaders want people to do this because this is both a source of innovative ideas and a motivation for change. When people create new ideas that excite them they become motivated to change things.

Whole-system conversations can include formal events, such as:

- project groups
- large group events
- conferences
- e-chat rooms.

They can include informal events, such as parties, networks and coffee rooms. The hope is similar in all – for like-minded people to spark off each other, generate new ideas and then try them out.

Whole-system conversations are helped by learning spaces, where participants reflect on their own real-life work, listen to the ideas of others and create new ideas that are a bit of both. Committee meetings can be learning spaces, but more commonly they operate in ways that reinforce the status quo. (You may be able to change this in the committee meetings you attend by using some of the ideas in this book. Be brave!)

Networks help whole-system conversations to take place between organisations. Key ideas generated in one place can be considered in other places. For example, successful audits can be showcased, and workshops can consider contentious issues for policy.

Relationships developed between disciplines and organisations can result in shared leadership for co-ordinated change. Feedback to everyone of progress provokes new ideas and understanding.

Implications for the clinical encounter

Encounters between clinician and patient can avoid being a one-way diagnosis of problems by developing a conversation approach. One approach has been described as 'narrative based',[17] clarifying and developing a patient's story.

Implications for running organisations and crafting policy

Committee meetings can become places where people learn. A listening, reflective and enquiring attitude is needed.

Implications for yourself

You can encourage whole-system conversations by building in feedback or communication loops between the groups to which you relate. For example, you can:

- send a regular e-mail to your constituents asking for their views about next steps, then feed back what has happened as a result, inviting further comment
- invite colleagues on your committee who also sit on other groups to talk for five minutes about shared areas of interest, or different ways of doing things.

Develop networks of high-performing teams

Trusted teams are the antidote to loneliness, and the source of power to act. You will need to nurture a number of teams to achieve your short- and long-term goals. Each team must have enough opportunity to develop its shared purpose. Members must know what to expect from each other. You will need teams of varying life-spans. They will not all be permanent. You will need the following.

- Teams that you call 'home' – where you feel you belong and are valued for your idiosyncrasies and what you contribute to team life as well as for your personal skills.
- Teams to complete different aspects of your work.
- Teams that more loosely connect different worlds of knowledge so you can open out conversations when the time is right.

At various times you may need to build these teams from scratch, then develop them as high-performing teams. Later you may come to see the individuals as friends. This is a healthy development. But remember to continue to appreciate and nurture them, and notice how they grow. It is very easy to take for granted those closest to you, to undervalue those who are most important to you, and to forget that people change.

The teams need to reflect as far as possible the diversity of perspectives from the whole system you are working with, even bits of it that seem alarming and alien. Different team members can therefore provide insight into how different constituencies think and feel in response to a change initiative (this will feel uncomfortable at times – it is much easier to invite people with whom you get on, and who 'see things your way'). These new colleagues will help to access people at appropriate times.

Regular communication with your teams is essential; this keeps everyone motivated to achieve your shared goals. Action plans need to be negotiated, documented and later checked for completion; this gives confidence in progress and in each others' skills. Protected time is needed for face-to-face meetings to revisit shared vision, and to identify new problems and new possibilities. This helps to keep the whole group together and air disagreements in private. An image or symbol that all agree summarises your shared identity helps all to quickly reconnect with your shared history.

Implications for the clinical encounter

Every person you encounter is potentially a team member, including patients in a consulting room. Being alert to this potential will help you to see them as full of potential, as partners rather than 'patients'. It will remind you to invest time and energy in building relationships.

Implications for running organisations and crafting policy

PCOs need to develop skilled and trusted teams and inter-organisational networks. These can often be done in everyday work. Cross-portfolio team-working can be developed systematically.

Implications for yourself

You need different teams for different purposes. You can plan their development in preparation for the challenges around the corner. You need to be a good team player in all aspects of your life, and, as a leader, you must at times allow your teams to support you.

Exercises

Reflect on what you think is good leadership

Bring to mind a change situation where you were impressed by what the change agent did. What did they do that impressed you? Write down what you think this says about how you think about leading change. Write down other ways of leading change. Write the strengths and weaknesses of each approach.

Design your personal development plan as a leader of whole-system change

Read the summaries at the beginning of all the chapters. Identify things that you need to prioritise for your own development.

Use the 'Things you can do to help the story evolve'

Read each of the four 'Things you can do . . .' above and decide which is most relevant to your present needs. Write your personal response to this. Include the ideas it brings up for you and what you can practically do. Then do it, and reflect on what you have learnt. Write it as an essay for your portfolio of learning.

Devise a rapid appraisal

Consider a situation you are trying to understand. Write down your present understanding of it. Use one of the techniques from Chapter 14 – a brainstorm, hexagons, mind-map or nominal grouping – to generate a list of people concerned with the issue. Make sure that this includes people outside your immediate field of view but relevant to successful change. To understand the situation quickly consider: (a) What literature will you read and why? (b) Who from your stakeholder list will you interview and what questions will you ask? (c) What situations will you observe and for what will you be looking? Then do it. Write down your new understanding of the situation.

Consider your preparedness to use whole-system interventions

Read the models in Chapter 15. Consider whether you and the people you work with are ready to try one of these. Design a whole-system event that you could practically operate with a trusted team. Do it. Write down what you have learned about facilitating whole-system events, and what you would do differently next time.

Identify your teams

Write down a list of the different teams to which you belong. Describe the purpose of each. Stand back and look at them as a whole, looking for duplications and weak links. How many of them could facilitate a learning space? How are you going to increase their abilities? Are there any teams that you need but are missing? Make a plan to develop any missing teams.

Revisit your case study

Re-read your previous plans about leading your chosen case study. Reflect first on how this chapter affirms what you were already planning. Reflect on what new insights the chapter has given you about an effective approach. In particular:

- Have you recognised that your situation includes a web of relationships that will affect how things go? Have you considered mapping these, or undertaking a rapid appraisal?
- Does your plan bring relevant stakeholders into the conversation? Does it include the creation of learning spaces where people can consider the implications of different courses of action, and then transfer this learning to other places? Have you identified facilitators for these?
- Have you identified a need for high-performance multi-disciplinary teams and have you plans to build them? What are you going to do about your own need for personal balance?
- Have you gained the support you need to achieve what you want and to protect you from nasty surprises? Will you be able to achieve three or more cycles of enquiry and action? Will you be able to access the right data at the right times?
- And what about the long term? Do you have plans to develop a sustainable infrastructure to support reflective practice and systems thinking, beyond your present brief? Are you thinking about ways to embed multi-disciplinary learning spaces that connect throughout the whole system over a variety of issues?

References

1 Kolb D (1984) *Experiential Learning*. Prentice Hall, Englewood Cliffs, NJ.
2 Argyris C and Schon DA (1977) *Organizational Learning: a theory of action perspective*. Addison-Wesley, New York.
3 Reason P (1994) Three approaches to participative inquiry. In: N Denzin and Y Lincoln (eds) *Handbook of Qualitative Research*. Sage, Thousand Oaks, CA.
4 Sainsbury P and Dowrick C (1995) Vision workshops – a planning tool for general practice. *Education in General Practice*. 6: 62–8.
5 Brandes D (1982) *Gamester's Handbook Two*. Hutchinson, Tiptree.
6 Kaagan SS (1999) *Leadership Games*. Sage, Thousand Oaks, CA.
7 Passmore W, Bunker BB, Jacobs R, Dannesmiller K, Alban B, Axelrod D *et al.* (1992) Large group interventions. *Journal of Applied Behavioral Science*. 28.
8 Stanley I, Al Shehr A and Thomas P (1993) Developing organisational vision in general practice. *BMJ*. **307**: 101–3.
9 Spratley J (1991) *Disease Prevention and Health Promotion in Primary Care*. Health Education Authority, London.
10 Spratley J (1991) *Joint Planning for the Development and Management of Disease Prevention and Health Promotion Strategies in Primary Care*. Health Education Authority, London.
11 Pratt J, Gordon P and Plamping D (1999) *Working Whole Systems: putting theory into practice in organisations*. King's Fund, London.
12 Benedict BB and Alban B (1997) *Large Group Interventions – Engaging the Whole System for Rapid Change*. Jossey-Bass, San Francisco, CA.
13 Attwood M, Pedler M, Pritchard S and Wilkinson D (2003) *Leading Change – A Guide to Whole System Working*. Policy Press, Abingdon.

14 Annett H and Rifkin S (1988) *Improving Urban Health. Guidelines for rapid appraisal to assess community needs. A focus on health improvements for low-income urban areas.* Liverpool School of Tropical Medicine, Liverpool.

15 Armson R, Ison RL, Short L, Ramage M and Reynolds M (2005) *Rapid institutional appraisal* (personal communication).

16 Patton MQ (1980) *Qualitative Evaluation and Research Methods.* Sage, Newbury Park, CA.

17 Launer J (2002) *Narrative-based Primary Care. A practical guide.* Radcliffe Medical Press, Oxford.

Chapter 5

Helping people to enquire and learn together

Summary

Leaders create 'learning spaces' – places where groups of people learn from and with each other, and develop collaborative enquiries – research and audit. This results in a better understanding of each other's contexts, and a growing sense of shared identity.

Listening to others (and to yourself) involves hearing both the words used and things that are not put into words. You need to respond to both. Responding in ways that the other cannot follow may make them feel that you are not listening.

Having identified the relevant stakeholders and understood something of their concerns it helps to bring them together at a 'whole-system event'. This is a learning space where people from all relevant perspective learn from and with each other, agree shared vision, and contribute to fashioning next steps.

At the event, moving backwards and forwards between small group discussions and large group plenary sessions helps to produce creative energy and also keep a sense of the whole group identity. Commitment is sought from all to engage in three connected cycles of reflection and action. The first cycle is concerned with establishing what is; the second with gaining a set of different insights into other ways of doing things; the third with developing policy to sustain a new integrated way of doing things. Each cycle includes a whole-system event where the evolution of the whole story is assessed.

Learning involves reflection – a process of reflecting experiences and ideas against other experiences and ideas. This produces new understandings. New understandings open the way for new ways of doing things – innovation.

This is the (Kolb) cycle of adult learning where theory and practice are made relevant to each other through experimentation and reflection.[1] The 'audit cycle' and 'action research' cycle[2] are also intended to be cycles of learning. Single-loop learning (Chapter 2) involves asking yourself if the words and ideas you use (theories) are the best ways to describe the world you experience. And if they are not, what words and ideas would be more true to your experience? Double-loop learning requires new insights, achieved by exposing yourself to new experiences and new ideas, and combining this with careful observation of what you can see, and listening to what you can hear.

Listening carefully involves paying attention to both the words people use and also to other signals they give without words. It also requires feedback to people so they know that you have listened. This serves both to check that you have heard correctly and also encourages them to elaborate to gain a fuller under-standing. People will feel that you are not listening if you fail to give this feedback in a way that they can relate to. Responding in ways that make people feel understood requires considerable skill.

Health care systems need multi-disciplinary learning. This gives participants windows into important experiences and ideas that are difficult to appreciate merely from the written word. It can provide a bridge whereby learning in one place or discipline is made accessible to others. It can challenge assumptions, open eyes to damaging behaviour and develop team skills. It can also remind you that you are working for the same goals as others, most of whom you do not know.

Multi-disciplinary learning can feel threatening or enjoyable depending on how safe participants feel. At its best it motivates and stretches participants, and builds high-performing teams. At its worst it precipitates posturing, blaming and superficial conversations that skirt around the real issues. At its best it describes a 'learning organisation', or a 'learning community'. These are discussed in Chapter 13.

In Chapter 3 I summarise Senge's five disciplines to lead a learning organ-isation. This is a set of disciplines not for dominating and controlling others, but for 'approaching one's life as a creative work, living life from a creative as opposed to a reactive viewpoint.'[3] It is a set of disciplines which underpin listening, reflection and rigorous enquiry.

Effective group learning needs careful planning (Chapter 16). Common things that obstruct learning are individuals who dominate, defensive behaviour and 'group-think'. Ways to deal with these include reframing accusations as ques-tions, putting issues to the whole group and frank one-to-one conversations. Techniques such as small-group–large-group iterations, games and 'time out' can often prevent polarisations. The further apart people are, the more difficult it is to get them to accept that they may be able to learn from others. The closer people are, the more difficult it is to explore new territory. The skilled facilitator has an array of techniques to deal with both.

Experienced facilitators can make their role seem easy. Don't be fooled – facilitating ways forwards in the midst of complex interactions and entrenched views is highly skilled work. Facilitators belong to the same breed as diplomats, peace-keepers and marriage guidance counsellors. They are considered irrelev-ant when everything is running smoothly. They are in the firing line when things are not.

Facilitators use techniques that help participants to recognise that they are part of multiple ongoing stories, and are only at the 'centre' of their own life story. Their insights are valuable, but they are not the only insights. Techniques to see things from other perspectives include role-play, goldfish bowls and scenario planning (Chapter 17). Mind-maps, brainstorms and nominal grouping help to connect one insight and another (Chapter 14). Facilitating self-organisation in a learning event enables participants to create groupings of their own choosing. This is helpful because it appeals directly to their self-interest, including their motivations for learning and action. Educational methods such as 'open space'[4] do this in a formal way (Chapter 15). Coffee rooms, corner shops and parties do this informally.

Choose your case study: developing shared plans for action

An introduction to this section can be found at the start of Part II.

Choose one of the following case studies and bear it in mind as you read the chapter. Choose one that is close to your own situation. These are the same cases described in each chapter of Part II so you may like to look back to see the story so far. Write down your initial ideas about how to manage the situation. Review these at the end of the chapter to see if your ideas have changed as a result of reading the chapter.

Developing a general practice: a small enterprise

You have impressed people with your ability to get things done. You have set up a personal appraisal system that you hope will develop your teams. You have employed someone to solve computer problems that have been preventing accurate data gathering. You hear most staff say that change is not possible. They say, 'We always start off enthusiastic then everything goes pear-shaped', or, 'It's all a good idea but we never have the time to follow through'. However, they have expressed a need for regular team meetings. But they have also expressed anxiety about the confrontational meeting style that they have experienced from some of the practitioners.

Your initial work identifies primary care professionals from other organisations who want to develop better relationships with the practice as an extended primary care team. They include a health visitor, two district nurses, a community psychiatric nurse and the co-ordinator of elderly services. You have identified people from several disciplines (receptionists, administrators, practice nurses, health visitors and GPs) who you sense may be able to develop the kind of leadership you think the organisation needs. Some were interested in the project you wanted to progress.

To score well in the new GP contract there is an urgent need to do many things at the same time. You recognise a need to make recording of patient data by clinicians more consistent, to have access to data about childhood immunisations done by health visitors in the community hospital, and to establish protocols for things such as disease and data management.

You decide to hold a meeting for the extended team members to hear their views and help to build a plan to move things forward.

Describe what you would do in this meeting to help people learn from and with each other, and to develop a shared plan.

Developing a community hospital: an institution

Your initial work identifies discontent among health visitors and district nurses. They feel that they are being pushed out of the community hospital, and that their views are not being heard. They also complain about the rudeness of some senior clinicians, who have been particularly vocal in the debate about reorganisation of the hospital. They say that this has upset several people and gets in the way of open discussions.

You hear from some GPs that their overwhelming workload and lack of places to think through issues has prevented a consensus developing among local GPs about the future of the hospital.

You hear from consultants their irritation at the slowness of progress and with GPs who do not turn up for meetings.

Several community groups had previously campaigned to keep the hospital open when its closure was suggested. Now the same groups are threatening to campaign through the newspapers because of what they see as a change from the idea of a holistic community hospital to an outpost of the teaching hospital.

Many do not know of the feasibility plan, or believe that it has been manipulated behind closed doors. You have identified a few people from different disciples who can see how complex things are. You think that they might be able to provide leadership for the whole initiative. You explored with them future potential and they expressed a need for regular open planning meetings, but also some anxiety that these will become confrontational and chaotic. You decide to host a stakeholder conference for different groups to air their views and help to build a plan to move things forward.

Describe what you would do in this meeting to help people learn from and with each other and develop a shared plan.

Developing primary care in localities

Your initial work identifies large numbers of priorities for your locality. You fed this information back to all GPs, nurses and practice managers, and asked them to further prioritise them.

The top priorities are the development of new models of intermediate care for diabetes and a redesign of mental health services. People were saying that to deal effectively with both of these there was a need to use existing resources better.

GPs thought that it took too long for a patient to see a psychiatrist and felt insufficiently supported in the mental health work they do. There was also anger that plans for the local community hospital seemed to have ignored requests for GP direct-access beds, and there was a perceived takeover of the community hospital plans by hospital consultants and the private sector.

You hear many people express a need for regular open meetings, but also anxiety about this because previous attempts at open meetings had resulted in nice-sounding ideas that were not followed through. Nevertheless, the locality steering group asks you to arrange an open meeting to help a diversity of people to contribute to next steps.

Describe what you would do in this meeting to help people learn from and with each other, and to develop a shared plan.

An image of a teacher: Paulo Friere

'Adult learning principles' underpin modern approaches to learning. This emphasises learning from experience.[5] It is curious to call this form of learning 'adult' because this is the way that children learn. The word *pedagogy* – the science of teaching – comes from the Greek words *pais* (boy) and *agogos* (to guide). Children naturally form ideas about the world from their experiments and experiences, helped by the words, concepts and theories given by those around them. Adult learning principles do the same, challenging us to see the world with less certainty and with more enquiry. Educationalists carry these ideas into classrooms throughout the world, producing an international network of leaders for learning.

The word *teacher* is insufficient for this understanding of learning. It carries connotations of giving and receiving knowledge. It comes from the Anglo-Saxon word *taecan* (to show, present or point out). Adult learning principles are concerned less with pointing things out, and more with helping people to find things out for themselves. This requires a learning environment – where it is easy to trust others, to reflect critically and listen, and to take risks by challenging the assumptions of yourself and others. It is less didactic (giving answers), and more Socratic (asking questions).

The origins of adult learning principles lie in the concept of 'empowerment learning', envisaged by Friere when working with the poor in Brazil.[6] He invited them to look at images of everyday situations and describe what they could see that was meaningful to them. Then he asked them what they would like to change and how they would do it.

This approach helped the poor people to step out of their usual ways of seeing insurmountable problems and see new potential in everyday situations. It challenged their assumptions that they could do nothing, and instead identified large numbers of practical things they could do. The empowering nature of these methods, and their ability to cause quick and relevant learning has resulted in their use in many developing world countries.[7] It reveals that change is possible, and what people must do to bring it about. It is empowering. It can be fun. It can transform organisations and systems. Friere was a real-life Mary Poppins.

Pause

In what ways are you a facilitator of learning for the people with whom you work?

A model that connects individual and team learning with action for change

This model is presented in two ways: (Figure 5.1) from the perspective of one learner or organisation; and (Figure 5.2) from the perspective of those leading whole-system learning and change.

From the perspective of one individual learner or organisation

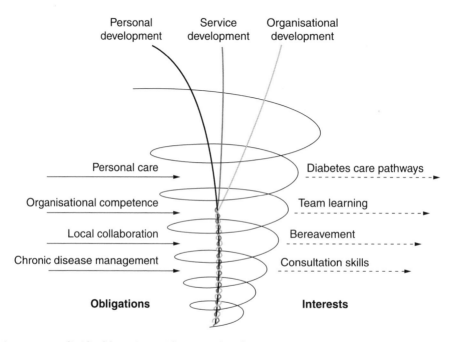

Figure 5.1 Individual learning with action for change.

The spirals of learning show that you revisit the same learning and change issues at different levels of complexity. For example, one year you may do something within your own team, the following year in the locality, and, later, on a bigger stage.

The solid arrows leading into the learning spirals represent your obligations – the certain side of the equation. The dotted arrows represent your multiple interests – any of which could be developed further. Both sides pose challenges for learning and change. Your task is for you and your team to find a good fit between your multiple obligations and interests which also helps to develop something practical for the whole service.

For example, you may be obliged to record which patients have severe mental illness, and you may have a personal interest in bereavement. A team discussion about obligations and interests in mental health might reveal that everyone is concerned about the poor services for those who are dying. A project to improve these services may allow many people to pursue related interests in synchrony and also improve mental illness monitoring through heightened awareness of mental health issues. The overall result is a weaving together of personal, service and organisational needs, allowing yourself and your team to grow at the same time.

From the perspective of those leading whole-system learning and change

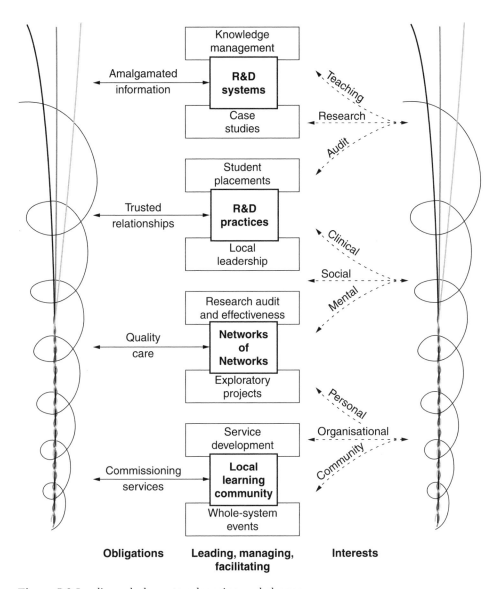

Figure 5.2 Leading whole-system learning and change.

Different individuals and organisations have different obligations and interests. Your task is to produce coalitions of interest from these to lead projects. You want to integrate the projects to move forwards the whole story, rather than merely those involved – perhaps by simultaneously developing diabetes information, diabetes audit and diabetes clinics.

The central part of the model shows mechanisms to integrate different initiatives. They involve leadership from systems, organisations, networks and localities:

- **R&D systems** – these include 'knowledge management' systems which help to make sense of a variety of information that can build up a rich local case study. Computer decision support, feedback of amalgamated data from relevant databases, evidence-based guidelines, public health statistics, websites, conclusions from whole-system events and maps of local services all contribute to R&D systems.
- **R&D practices** – A R&D practice differs from a traditional research practice by becoming skilled at facilitating integrated efforts for enquiry and quality, as well as being able to pose important research questions and generate reliable answers to them. It includes a multi-disciplinary team that takes a local leadership role for research and audit, and local reflection on the practical implications of these. They help generate new knowledge about primary care, and support developments that will lead to quality integrated primary health care. They relate to those leading service commissioning and reserve redesign and encourage them to consider a breadth of perspective. They relate to a local network of interested organisations and individuals, and encourage them to create a culture of reflection and enquiry. They relate to universities, and provide a route for them to pilot new initiatives, facilitate student placements and recruit to research projects.
- **Networks of networks** – these connect multiple networks for research, audit and quality. They can bring together people with different insights to support local developments. Project groups, priority action groups, local implementation teams and primary care research networks should all have pathways into networks.
- **Local learning community** – this is a broad coalition of stakeholders united in wishing to integrate local efforts for health. They use whole-system events to develop co-ordinated action plans for service improvements. Shared leadership facilitates ongoing feedback from multiple insights to retain a synchrony of effort.

Examples of learning spaces in primary care

Externally facilitated team learning

A multi-disciplinary team (Liverpool) facilitated in-practice multidisciplinary reflection and action in a model of group learning termed a 'Roadshow'. It lasted 90 minutes. The home team included five to ten people (usually doctors and nurses from the extended primary care team). The visiting team included facilitators who reflected the disciplines of the home team.

The home team chose the topic, for example their diabetic or immunisation clinics.[8] One person from the home team prepared data about the issue. The visiting team followed a semi-structured format that clarified the purpose, explored roles, problems and solutions, and helped the home team to create an action plan.

Merely airing the views of other team members frequently revealed systemic problems that no one was aware of (for example, duplication of recording). Participants frequently found it energising because they came to realise how much good work was being done. They were also able to produce their own plan for change, which was willingly embraced, solving problems that were concerning everyone.

Internally facilitated team learning

A general practice (London) held two in-practice educational meetings each month, both relating to the same theme. At the 'educational meeting', a member of staff presented an update, or a new project. At the 'quality meeting' three or four audits, pilot projects or significant events were presented. A different multiprofessional group led each month. The summaries documented the development of the practice as a whole.

Locality multi-disciplinary workshops

A multi-disciplinary facilitation team (Liverpool) facilitated a monthly locality workshop of 90 minutes where practitioners presented new ideas to each other and debated the relevance of the idea in other places.[9] After a presentation lasting 15 minutes small groups discussed (for 45 minutes) the relevance of the idea to them, and ways in which the idea could be modified to better effect.

Feedback often revealed similar thinking in all parts of the room, and this led to a room consensus about what could be done to improve things. This gave impetus to projects that went on to have an impact throughout the city, and at times nationally. One of many examples was the recognition that different district nurses treated leg ulcers in different ways, and that there were no agreed guidelines for optimal treatment. This led to new city-wide protocols for management, and a national conference on leg ulcer care which affected nursing practice nationwide.

GP updating meetings

A monthly 90-minute educational meeting for GPs which included a presentation from a hospital specialist (Liverpool). It started with a brainstorm of what things were of particular interest to the participants. This list commonly included things that the specialist had not intended to include, so they altered their plan there and then to address these concerns. This often resulted in animated two-way discussions that made the meetings fun and creative.

Interactive newsletter

A general practice (London) produced a quarterly two-page newsletter for patients. The second page included questions about things of contemporary interest. The first page summarised the responses from the previous newsletter, explaining how the practice has responded to these, and posing new issues for consideration by patients. The sequence of first pages documented the evolution of the practice over time.

Things you can do to help people to enquire and learn together

Facilitate whole-system events

Sooner or later you will need to get a broad group of stakeholders in the same room to hear each other's perspectives, agree shared purpose and devise practical next steps.

Getting the right people to attend requires: (a) an invitation from those perceived to be leaders in this context; (b) an urgent or tricky question that attracts their interest; (c) a sense of confidence and competence that this meeting will move things forward; and (d) making it easy for people to attend.

At the meeting you may have to deal with entrenched positions, anger and impossible expectations of what can be achieved. Good facilitation will largely avoid these and lead to a description of what is known and what is not, what is agreed and what is not, a commitment to keep in the conversation, and practical ways forwards that build relationships and skills, as well as produce valuable outputs.

An exercise in backwards mapping (Chapter 6) helps to work out what amount of time is needed for each part of the meeting.

A summary of the story so far is often a good start, with a restatement of the question to be explored. Small-group–large-group iterations (Chapter 16) allow people to generate energy by talking directly to others, and also hold together the whole group. Keeping plenary feedback to a minimum avoids losing energy.

The meeting should help participants to step out of the things that are immediately concerning them, to see other things of relevance to which they may have become blind through over-familiarity. It takes people on a journey, and brings them back to almost exactly where they were at the beginning, but with new eyes. Role-play, goldfish bowls and scenario planning can help people to see with different eyes (Chapter 17).

Other techniques that may help include brainstorming to bring into view interconnected factors (Chapter 14). Ground rules and energisers help participants to feel safe to express opinions (Chapter 16).

If things go well, participants come to see the relevance of their own insights to those of others. This can feel invigorating but also challenging when participants recognise that they need to change their own behaviour.

The process can be emotionally demanding for the facilitators. You are always working with the energies within the group as it explores questions, rather than providing answers. You have to stimulate creative thinking without too much conflict. You may have to help the group stay with uncomfortable feelings for a while. You may have to intervene in a direct way to address misunderstandings.

Implications for the clinical encounter

You can make the consulting room a 'whole-system event' where a patient makes sense of different aspects of their health.

Implications for running organisations and crafting policy

Regular whole-system events help to harness the energies of different people. Practitioners and managers need to become skilled at facilitating them.

Implications for yourself

It is easy to neglect this process for yourself and your teams. Your yearly calendar should include times when people from the different parts of your personal and professional lives can re-find a sense of shared story.

Institutionalise cycles of enquiry

You may have agreed with your stakeholders to lead three connected cycles of reflection and action (see the model in Chapter 2). It may help you to think of the first cycle as being concerned with 'establishing what is'; the second with gaining a set of different 'insights into new ways of doing things'; the third with exploring how those insights can be brought together to 'fashion policy to sustain a new way of doing things'.

Each cycle involves gathering data and considering its meaning in the light of the experiences of the stakeholders. The more you can involve them in the process the better. This is a version of participatory action research – stakeholders are involved at all stages of an enquiry.[10]

An exploratory 'pilot' project is a useful focus for gathering data because it gives people a chance to experience what a new way of doing things would feel like. This 'learning by doing' allows a participant to see potential that is invisible in the data that is generated. It is important that people learn from these exploratory projects, and change the plans accordingly. They should not be seen merely as a prelude to larger implementation.

This process can also be seen as three cycles of 'audit'. The audit cycle is a cycle of learning. Data gathering without learning is not audit. The audit cycle requires stakeholders to agree in advance what data are to be gathered and why. It requires that they later reflect on its meaning and make changes that are later audited.

Audit does not merely measure quantitative standards. It can include any rigorous examination of quality, including qualitative and participatory enquiries. As with research, the combination of quantitative, qualitative and participatory approaches helps to explore the depth of issues and find the best ways forward (Chapter 11). Quantitative measurement of standards encourages single-loop learning (Chapter 2) concerned with slight adjustments, rather than with facilitating more fundamental change (Chapter 13).

Audit, in the sense I am using it, can be the same activity as research. Audit generates knowledge for local learning, and research generates knowledge of more generalisable value. As with research, rigorous data gathering is needed. As with research, the aim is to provide reliable answers to important questions.

By calling these cycles of reflection and enquiry 'audit' you have the advantage of connecting your work as a leader of change with existing systems of audit support, refocusing them to support co-ordinated efforts for whole-system change and leadership development. Emphasising three connected cycles rather than one shows how to create focus within complex adaptivity.

Linking the idea of these cycles of reflection and enquiry with research helps practitioners of each to move between them. It helps to use research tools and techniques for audit purposes, thereby increasing the rigour of an enquiry.

You can set up support for local audit groups to work with research teams. This could develop synchronous quantitative and qualitative research and audit. Ongoing cycles of enquiry can increase recruitment to a research project,[11] as well as increase local research capacity.

Implications for the clinical encounter

You can encourage patients to undertake their own enquiries about their health. For example by keeping a diary of symptoms, exploring self-help opportunities through the internet or by experimenting with different treatments.

Implications for running organisations and crafting policy

Research and audit functions could be synchronised within PCOs, practice-based commissioning, unscheduled care services, and other organisations that have a remit for whole geographical areas. This could connect efforts for research, audit, leadership and organisational development, making efficient use of resources.

Implications for yourself

You, too, need to be skilled at rigorous enquiries, and use these to learn.

Surface mental models

There is a joke about an optimistic man who was given a heap of horse manure for his birthday – he scrabbled within it, saying, 'There's got to be a horse in here somewhere'.

He is demonstrating a mental model – a 'deeply ingrained assumption, general-isation, picture or image that influences how we understand the world and how we take action'.[3] The mental model of the optimistic man may reflect his general attitude towards all things, or it may be an expectation of a specific context. Either way it represented a prejudgement about what to expect, that led to behaviour that was 'logical' or 'natural' only to him.

All people use these subconscious ideas. They lead them to anticipate what will happen as the result of their actions and those of others. They frame what they can see in situations, and how they will respond. If someone has a dominant mental model that imagines change to result from overcoming resistance, they will use force. If they imagine that change results from resolving misunderstand-ings, they will use education. If they imagine that change results from ownership of a change process they will encourage participation. A mental model filters out from complex wholes those aspects that fit with that preferred way of looking. They colour every aspect of thinking and action.

Mental models are powerful determinants of how people behave – more powerful than what they say. There are long-held habits and not easy to change. They are theories-in-use, rather than espoused theories of action.[12] Knowing what they are in others helps you to know what to expect from them. Knowing your own helps to know what to expect of yourself. It can also help you to move deliberately between different mental models, depending on the need.

Techniques that reveal mental models include word association, structured feedback from critical friends, imaginary journeys, mind-maps, identifying with images, attitude cards, role-play, goldfish bowls and personal drawings of where participants see themselves in respect of an evolving story. Some of these techniques are described in Part IV. Each holds up a mirror to the face of a learner to see him or herself as others see them.

Argyris teaches a systematic way to surface mental models.[13] He invites learners to describe an organisational problem, and to imagine a conversation with a key person about how to improve things. On the right hand side of a paper the interviewer (the learner) writes what they would say and what they believe the other would say in response, then their response to their response, continuing this scenario for a couple of pages. Afterwards, in the left-hand column they write ideas and feelings that they would not communicate for one reason or another within this imaginary dialogue. Reviewing this work with colleagues gives insight to mental models of themselves and others on both sides of the paper.

Changing mental models requires more than knowing about them. They are ingrained habits, comparable with addictions, and a part of someone's sense of self. Learning to change them requires discipline, persistent friendly support and enough stress-free space to give it a go.

Implications for the clinical encounter

Medical training leads to a dominant mental model of linearity (Chapter 11). This sees diseases as discrete entities and laboratory science as the highest form of enquiry. Being effective at whole-person care requires you to also use non-linear mental models.

Implications for running organisations and crafting policy

Bureaucratic organisations encourage linear 'hard systems thinking'[14] and compartmentalised effort through the image of organisations as machines.[15] Other mental models, such as brains, cultures or organisms,[15] encourage 'soft systems thinking'[14] and complex adaptivity, which are more appropriate to learning organisations. Organisations need a balance of different mental models, and to use them well.

Implications for yourself

To be an effective leader you need to understand the mental models that largely inform your thinking and actions, and be able to use a selection. You need to be able to surface them in others, and help them to change them.

See things through other eyes

Whole-system change needs people from throughout the system to be mindful of the effect their actions have on others. When you understand what it is like from someone else's perspective you become better able to adapt your own behaviour to be complementary to theirs. This empathy allows you to feel on the same side rather than an adversary. This helps to build trusted relationships and promotes team-working.

As with everyone else, you will largely be blind to the effect your past experiences have on the way you interpret the world, and on the effect you have on others. It is easy, and common, to blame and misrepresent others, when the 'fault' lies with the accuser for failing to understand the other; or worse – when the accuser is merely projecting their own traits (Chapter 8).

Role-play, video analysis, goldfish bowls and feedback from trusted friends can all help to see things the way others do. Some of these techniques are described in Chapter 17.

Finding out about different people's learning styles or learning about Myers Briggs personality-type indicators could both help you to become more aware of yourself and to see better through other's eyes.

Listening carefully to what people say gives clues to what it is like from their perspective, both what they say in words and what they say in actions. Repeating back to people what they have said, opening the way to explore other things and giving thoughtful responses can develop trust sufficient to explore more difficult things. Responding to something other than what someone has said, or telling people that they are wrong, can both make people feel that they are not heard and you are not on their side.

Dealing promptly with problems as people perceive them builds trust. Here, you are demonstrating that you have not only heard but are acting on what you have heard. More specifically, it becomes clear to them that you are acting in their interests. Trust makes it easier for someone to contemplate change.

Dealing well with misunderstandings can build trust. Misunderstandings about fact can often be resolved by looking at the facts together. Misunderstandings about expectations can be helped by ground rules.

Sometimes different interpretations arise from things deeper than misunderstandings. For example, team members may have fundamentally different ways of thinking about the task in hand. This can be very uncomfortable for the individuals concerned. The whole team may have to help move forwards in a positive way. Facilitation may be needed.

Implications for the clinical encounter

Being able to recognise that different people see the world quite differently is helpful to you as a practitioner. Your training will have taught you to value objective scientific evidence above other forms of evidence. This inhibits seeing things from other perspectives. Seeing things as others see them requires listening and reflection. It means valuing subjective truths as well as objective facts (Chapter 11). It means recognising the importance of the coherence of someone's story over any of these different kind of truths.

Implications for running organisations and crafting policy

Developing an organisational culture that values diversity will require widespread skills to see things through the eyes of others. Organisations will need to ensure that leaders throughout the organisation are skilled at leading techniques that help this.

Implications for yourself

You will need to show by example that you are able to appreciate other people's perspectives. You will need ways to manage your own anxieties that arise from trying to appreciate things that you do not agree with.

Exercises

Most of these exercises need to be done with a trusted team. Try inviting them to give you feedback about your performance.

Use the 'Things you can do to help people to enquire and learn together'

Read each of the four 'Things you can do . . .' above and decide which is most relevant to your present needs. Write your personal response to this. Include the ideas it brings up for you and what you can practically do. Then do it and reflect on what you have learnt. Make it into an essay to put into your portfolio of learning.

Devise a whole-system event

Devise one or more multi-disciplinary educational sessions that are relevant to your own work. Use the techniques described in Chapter 16. Facilitate and evaluate the session. If you enjoy it, consider undertaking a formal course on facilitating adult learning.

Engage your teams in ongoing cycles of enquiry

Consider each of your teams in turn. What ongoing meetings or projects are they involved in? What conversations external to their immediate concerns could they usefully have? How can you use their connections with other parts of the system, and develop their own skills of network operating.

Facilitate the surfacing of mental models

Within an educational meeting get participants to describe different metaphors for change. Ask them to reflect on what understandings are hidden in these metaphors, which ones they prefer, and why. Ask them which ones they identify with, and what this says about them.

Facilitate a role-play or goldfish bowl

Within an educational meeting facilitate a role-play or goldfish bowl as described in Chapter 17. Facilitate a discussion about how this helps participants to see things from other people's perspectives.

Draw your own life-line

Draw a life-line (Chapter 14). Stand back and look at this. Ask yourself what this says about who you are and how you want to develop.

Revisit your case study

Re-read your plans for your enterprise/institution/network to enable a variety of disciplines to contribute to a shared plan. Reflect first on how this chapter affirms what you were already planning. Reflect on what new insights the chapter has given you about an effective approach. In particular:

- Have you identified learning spaces where individuals and multi-disciplinary teams can engage at the level of their interests? Do you have ways for them to make connections between their personal development needs and those of their organisations and services? Are you nurturing these people so they will in time be able to devise and lead whole-system learning events?
- Did you feel confident to devise a whole-system event? How are you going to increase your knowledge and skills to make these effective learning occasions for all involved? Do you need to go on a teaching or group facilitation course, or experiment with more advanced applications of your existing skills?
- Are you aware of techniques that reveal the mental models of participants: structured feed-back from critical friends, imaginary journeys, mind-maps, identifying with images, role-play and personal drawings of where they see themselves in respect of an evolving story? Had you considered including these in your meeting?
- Are you aware of techniques that help people to see things through other people's eyes: role-play, video analysis, goldfish bowls and feedback from trusted friends? Had you considered including these in your meeting?

References

1 Kolb D (1984) *Experiential Learning*. Prentice Hall, Englewood Cliffs, NJ.
2 Weil S (1997) Postgraduate education and lifelong learning in public service organisations. Systematic practice and organisational learning as critically reflexive action research (CRAR). *Systematic Practice and Action Research*. **11**: 37–61.
3 Senge P (1993) *The Fifth Discipline*. Century Hutchinson, London.
4 Owen H (1997) *Open Space Technology – A User's Guide*. Berrett-Koehler, San Francisco, CA.
5 Knowles M (1980) *The Modern Practice of Adult Learning: from pedagogy to androgogy*. Cambridge Books, New York, NY.
6 Friere P (1970) *Pedagogy of the Oppressed*. Seabury Press, New York, NY.
7 Hope A, Timmel S and Hodzi C (1991) *Training for Transformation – A Handbook for Community Workers*. Mambo Press, Gweru.
8 Thomas P (1994) *The Liverpool Primary Health Care Facilitation Project 1989–1994*. Liverpool Family Health Services Authority, Liverpool.
9 Thomas P and Graver LD (1997) The Liverpool intervention to promote teamwork in general practice: an action research approach. In: EDS Pearson and J Spencer (eds) *Promoting Teamwork in Primary Care – A Research Based Approach*. Arnold, London.
10 Whyte WF (1991) *Participatory Action Research*. Sage, New York, NY.
11 Donovan J, Mills N, Smith M, Brindle L, Jacoby A, Peters T *et al.* (2002) Improving design and conduct of randomised controlled trials by embedding them in qualitative research: ProtecT (prostate testing for cancer and treatment) study. *BMJ*. **325**: 766–70.
12 Argyris C and Schon DA (1996) *Organizational Learning 2 – Theory, Method, and Practice*. Addison Wesley, Reading, MA.

13 Argyris C (1996) Skilled incompetence. In: K Starkey (ed) *How Organizations Learn.* International Thompson Publishing Company, London.
14 Checkland P (1995) *Systems Thinking, Systems Practice.* Wiley, Bath.
15 Morgan G (1997) *Images of Organisation.* Sage, Thousand Oaks, CA.

Chapter 6

Infrastructures that facilitate ongoing learning and change

Summary

Strategic coalitions and backwards mapping help people at the most peripheral places to have room to be creative.

System maps and timetables help people to navigate a system for themselves. They can also help to plan complex interventions. You can draw the system of concern on a flip chart to show the flow of people and data. This often reveals the lack of connection between one thing and another. When maps and timetables help people to make decisions for improvement they come to value them.

Networks facilitate cross-organisational learning and change when they create 'learning spaces'. Here, members of different organisations learn from and with others, and develop shared projects. Shared leadership can result. Building from this for the long term requires sustained high-level political support. Different networks can be connected at 'nodes'. These produce a network of networks which can help to integrate the effect of all involved.

The output from multiple connected networks can be kept manageable through gatekeepers at the nodes. Gatekeepers filter out useful ideas and help them to be accessed by others.

Whole-system events can cross-pollinate ideas between different networks and build a 'learning community'. Bringing together people and data from the same geographic area helps to build a rich picture of that area as well as build relationships. It can also result in combined research and audit projects, shared evaluation of complex interventions and shared training. Network infrastructure needs to be maintained after its immediate priority has been achieved. Like the tracks on which trains run, networks need to be maintained even when there is no traffic if they are to be ready to take advantage of later opportunities.

The technique of 'backwards mapping' helps to identify both what is realistic and what is enabling for others. This can be applied to devising plans, monitoring projects and accessing the right kind of data at the right times.

Leaders want innovation to happen throughout whole systems and not merely in local pockets. This can be achieved by applying the principles of multi-disciplinary learning, outlined in Chapter 5, to networks. A network is a group of people connected by a shared interest. Networks can help stimulate 'shared leadership' for learning and change between the organisations they connect.

Written papers, talks and conferences are the usual ways to transfer knowledge from one part of the system to another. These help large numbers of people to catch glimpses of innovative ideas. But it is a one-way passive activity that does little to create energy or broker the partnerships which are needed to turn ideas into action. Conversely, ongoing conversations between people who care about an issue can develop these conditions. Coalitions of interest can test out ideas and feed progress back at a later stage.

A good peer reviewing process helps to illustrate a successful conversation within a network. The network is the journal readership. Authors submit papers that they consider to contain important learning for others. Editorial gatekeepers reject some immediately (first feedback loop). Reviewers subject others to critical and supportive review. These comments are fed back to the authors (second feedback loop). If a paper is not accepted as it is, an author will reflect on the reviews and decide what to do next. This may include resubmission (third feedback loop), or submitting the paper to a journal with a different readership (moving to another system/network). The authors, editors and reviewers are all in different learning spaces which connect with feedback loops. Each takes their turn to reflect on the value of a paper as it is, and suggests how it could be made more relevant to the journal readership.

Network leaders must put in place these learning spaces and feedback loops. They must also make the whole system clear to its members. Networks can prevent overload by creating gate-keeping roles like the journal editors. This allows the filtering of useful ideas and making them accessible to other parts of the system. Take the example of clinical governance – a network of clinical governance leaders from different PCOs could filter their best audits and show-case them through a shared quarterly bulletin or annual conference, encouraging cross-PCO discussion about transferable lessons.

Multi-disciplinary conversations can be facilitated within conferences through workshops and discussions around a poster. Conferences can purposefully invite people from a variety of networks to cross-pollinate ideas. For example, a conference on diabetes care could plan participation of people from other clinical networks, workforce development and information technology (IT). Large-group techniques are particularly good at enabling meaningful conversations between many different constituencies.

A whole-system event can bring together people from the same geographic area. It will build relationships and also provide a rich picture of what is happening. It can spawn combined research or audit projects, shared evaluation of local services, local self-help groups and shared training courses. Crossover points, such as these annual meetings, are 'nodes' – places that connect different networks, different worlds of understanding.

A railway network shows how to facilitate the nodes in a complex of networks. Different travellers devise their journeys with maps and timetables. At the nodes (railway junctions) travellers choose to get on different trains, and strike up conversations with fellow travellers if the atmosphere allows. Deciding which train to get on and which travellers to talk to are helped by good information about the trains and the travellers. Facilitators will help people to listen to each other. The 'rule of two feet' forces people to take responsibility for their own navigation of the system – if you want to talk to someone else, just walk.

Leadership builds this infrastructure of communication and feedback.

Choose your case study: building infrastructures for ongoing learning and change

An introduction to this section can be found at the start of Part II.

Choose whichever of the following case studies is most like your own situation. These are the same cases described in each chapter of Part II, and you may like to look back to see how the story has unfolded so far. Write down your initial ideas about how to manage the situation. Review these at the end of the chapter to see if your ideas have changed as a result of reading the chapter.

Developing a general practice

Your whole-team meeting was a great success. It lasted a entire afternoon and took place in the practice. The multi-disciplinary team you nurtured devised a good programme for the event, helped by a professional facilitator. Almost everyone invited attended – 25 people. The presentations made by the practice leads for IT, clinical governance and reception were well received. The small group work produced a lot of ideas, and the whole meeting had an energising sense of a team waiting to fly.

You emerged from the meeting with commitment from three project groups to develop three projects: data managing systems; clinical governance systems; and systems to act on complaints. You called them 'project teams' but think of them as 'system redesign teams' to indicate that the practice gives them permission to suggest ways of redesigning their part of the system. They were asked to feedback at the next all-team meeting suggestions for pilot projects to move things forward. Each group arranged a time for their first meeting.

The team that devised the event was asked to also lead the next all-team meeting in three months' time and to oversee the whole initiative. It was called a 'steering group' but you think of it as the 'system transformation team' to imply that it is charged with facilitating transformation over time of the whole system. In addition, the clinical team agreed to a weekly meeting to discuss patients. Monthly meetings of the whole practice were planned to consider new issues. You wrote up the meeting and distributed the plan to everyone.

Within a month the warm glow had dissipated and the tasks seemed overly ambitious. Staff conflicts emerged as people expected a level of co-operation from colleagues that did not seem to happen. Two of the three groups postponed their first meeting. You were unable to find a time for the monthly team meeting because of the commitments of the various part-timers. At times it felt to you that everyone expected everything to change overnight but without any effort on their part. You felt that you were the only one who recognised that there had to be disciplined meetings and sustained effort. Six weeks later the atmosphere was poor. People started to blame you. You are feeling defensive.

Write down what you would do to overcome this setback, empower your project teams and help them to build their own networks.

Developing a community hospital

Your whole-system event was successful. It lasted a whole day and took place in a local hotel that offered a concessionary rate. The multi-disciplinary team you nurtured devised a good programme for the event, helped by an experienced facilitator who was recommended for this type of event. One hundred and fifty people attended, covering most of the groups you considered should be involved. Fifteen different community groups were represented. The initial four presentations gave complementary insights into the story so far and led to a robust exchange of views. The style of the chair gave confidence through a skilful combination of listening, determination to overcome obstacles and humour. This set the perfect base for the energising vision-setting exercise before lunch. Here multi-disciplinary groups of about eight people described: (a) what they would like to see in 10 years' time; (b) what streams of work should be developed to bring this about; and (c) what next steps were needed. The wall became papered with flip-chart paper. At the plenary session the facilitator invited snap-shot comments from the groups, which built up a convincing consensus about the long-term hopes for the hospital.

Some strongly held ideas emerged that gained agreement throughout the conference: a hope that the hospital would act as a focus to pull together, or point to, the large number of local services – medical, social, statutory and voluntary; a hope to retain overnight beds and the operating theatre; and a concern about the inadequacy of care for the elderly and mentally unwell. The rest of the day involved a sequence of small group workshops and short plenary feedback about these three issues.

The meeting ended with agreement to set up three multi-disciplinary project teams to explore these three areas in more depth and report back at the next whole-system event in six months' time. They were called 'project teams' but you think of them as 'system redesign teams' to indicate that they were given permission to suggest ways of redesigning their part of the system. The original team that designed the event was congratulated. It was asked to become a steering group to oversee the whole initiative. You think of it as a 'system transformation team' to imply that it was charged with facilitating transformation (over time) of the whole system. In addition, a project team of three, under your immediate direction, agreed to service the groups, to be a contact point for everyone and to organise the next event. You wrote up the meeting and distributed the plan to everyone.

The next week you were summoned to a meeting with a senior manager. There had been complaints about you from senior people in the health care system. You were accused of 'muddying the waters' and 'raising impossible expectations' from people who 'did not understand the financial realities'. You presented a confident exterior and gained agreement to continue. But inside you had your own doubts – was it really possible to hold all this together? Would it spiral out of control? Were those involved experienced enough to make progress fast enough? You are feeling defensive.

Write down what you would do to overcome this setback, empower your project teams and help them to build their own networks.

Developing primary care in localities

Your open meeting was eye-opening for everyone. Many participants were used to slow-moving committees that focused on medical concerns. This meeting was different – there was laughter, colour and many new ideas. Forty people attended a half-day meeting in a large room provided free at the local community hospital. It started a bit slowly, everyone sitting round a long boardroom-style table. People listened thoughtfully to an account of how the two priorities (mental health and diabetes) had emerged and agreed that they were important. The next exercise changed the entire mood of the meeting. The participants wrote on Post-Its (sticky paper squares) their personal opinions about what priorities had to be addressed (in blue pen) and what they would personally like to see done (in red pen). The point of the coloured pens was that political priorities are likely to indicate resources and personal interests are likely to indicate enthusiasm to take part. Then in groups of three or four the participants explained to each other why they thought these things. Then they stuck all the Post-Its on a large wall and everyone moved them around to form themes. The energy in this 'marketplace of ideas' was palpable, with laughter and multiple interactions in all parts of the room. People who you would never expect to warm to this sort of large-group technique spontaneously took roles. Some took a policing role making sure that the themes were not duplicated; others took a facilitating role, encouraging people to be more assertive about their ideas; others enthusiastically took to the task of forming themes.

Two people had been asked to feed back the information on the wall to the whole group. This revealed 20 different themes, of which two large ones were the previously identified issues of mental health and diabetes. A third large theme also emerged – the elderly. The group as a whole agreed that these three themes should be the focus of their next steps, and all themes should be written up for later consideration. The entire exercise lasted 45 minutes. The rest of the meeting was taken up by forming three multi-disciplinary groups to explore these three areas in more depth with the intention of reporting back at the next meeting in three months' time. They became called 'project teams', but you think of them as 'system redesign teams' to indicate that they were given permission to suggest ways of redesigning their part of the system. The steering group was congratulated and asked to oversee the whole initiative, with the next meeting in three months' time. You think of this group as a 'system transformation team' to imply that it was charged with facilitating transformation (over time) of the whole system. You wrote up the meeting and distributed the plan to everyone.

The three groups had their meetings within two months and you attended all of them, but several people did not attend, and the meetings produced little more than had the larger meeting. You started to suspect that everyone expected everything to be done by you. It was as though people were so used to one-off events they were not used to sustaining their own personal contribution when the spotlight was off them.

Write down what you would do to overcome this setback, empower your project teams and help them to build their own networks.

An image of inter-organisation innovation: a carnival

The Notting Hill Carnival, in north-west London, is one of the largest street parties in the world. It provides a useful image for health care about how to facilitate innovation at multiple levels when tens of thousands of people pursue different interests in different ways. The organising committee includes all perspectives of society – residents, police, artists, vendors . . . They are charged with the overall plan, and adapting this to the changing times. They are a 'transformation team' because they oversee the changing form of the whole event each year, including new themes, new routes and new rules of behaviour. They develop policies which consider both previous experience and new expectations. For example, when larger numbers are expected, or when there was violence in the previous year, the number of police increases.

But there are many innovations that have little to do with the committee. Live bands, piped music, dance troupes and food outlets have all been planned long in advance by others. Each has its own 'design team', concerned with the success of their individual concern. Each is given, or takes, space where they can do their thing, within an overall intention to create music and dance, and reach out to others with whom they would not ordinarily communicate. Each member of the enormous crowd organises him- or herself, helped by a map of the roads and the timetable of events; and helped by an army of police, carnival attendants and locals who know how to negotiate the back streets, and who join in the fun but mobilise quickly when trouble brews.

You can tell when things are going well because people spontaneously smile and laugh, and dance and sing. Everyone gives room to babies in prams, invites those who look lost to join in and helps to nip trouble in the bud. You can tell when things are going badly because people look tired and quiet, squashed or frightened. They look for ways to get out and become angry with those in their way.

The factors that help the Notting Hill Carnival to go well are things that help people to know where they are, and move to where they want to go and to play games with each other. Confusion and irritation comes when the parade goes in a way other than that indicated on the map, or when mounted police block the only exit. Certain behaviour precipitates the same behaviour in others: laughter and dance causes others to laugh and dance; anger and violence causes retreat and defence. Each group carves out a space for its creative interaction. Individuals move between these spaces causing dynamic and organic change in overall shape of the mass of people, all adapting to each other.

Pause

In what ways do you create a carnival atmosphere in your work?

A model of connected learning spaces

The model (Figure 6.1) describes things to consider when facilitating whole-system learning.

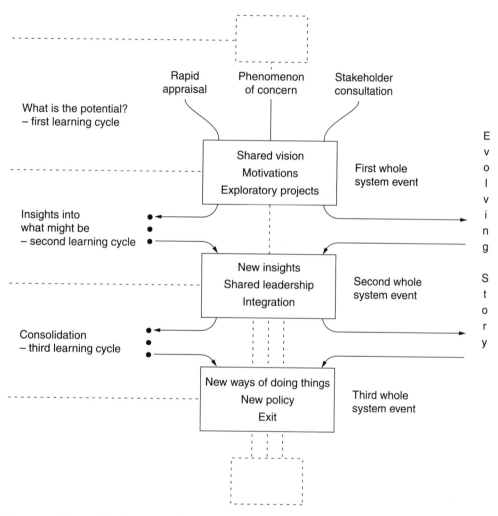

Figure 6.1 A model of connected learning spaces.

You must be clear about what story, phenomenon of concern or network of interests is concerned to decide what stakeholders to invite. The connected learning spaces are infrastructure to help develop the story that is shared by those who engage. The leaders 'hold the story'.

The spaces can be a series of whole-system events, team meetings or workshops to explore an emerging issue. They can be nodes which connect different geographical areas or portfolios of work. They can be the regular appearance of a journal. They must happen at predictable times and places so participants can choose when to engage. In each case you have in mind a long-term series of events with project and inquiry groups working in between.

You may wish to bunch events into threes in order to facilitate discrete stages within a longer-term journey. If you do this: the first event is largely concerned with establishing a shared understanding of what is the present situation and future potential as perceived by the stakeholders; the second event is largely concerned with gaining exploratory insights into this potential; and the third is largely concerned with developing policy to integrate and sustain progress of that stage.

A variety of data are needed for each learning space. These are needed to help participants to see what is the present state and future vision for their shared story, and what next steps are desirable. Data can come from a variety of research and audit projects – literature reviews, surveys, quantitative and qualitative studies, case studies, participatory research.

Examples of infrastructures that facilitate ongoing learning and change

The Liverpool Occupational Health Project

Patients in general practice waiting rooms were interviewed about their hazards at work. They fed back the information to practice teams and amalgamated it across the city. This initiative involved no payments to practitioners but involved almost half of the practices in the city. Important occupational health issues were identified, practitioners improved their skills at occupational health and a number of campaigns produced tangible successes.

Local multi-disciplinary facilitation teams

Four multi-disciplinary teams of local practitioners facilitated learning and communication within localities of the city (Liverpool).[1,2] Learning from different disciplines and practices was explored locally, and learning from this was shared across the city. The four teams greatly increased the ability of other groups to access general practice and facilitate locality innovation. It also provided a mechanism for city-wide dissemination of local innovation. They learnt the skills of whole-system leadership through a dedicated university certificate.

West London Research Network

At the annual conference of the West London Research Network (WeLReN) participants privately wrote on Post-Its (sticky squares) what they considered to be the research priorities for the year (using a blue pen for a development priority and a red pen if the writer was interested in the topic). The hundred or so participants moved these squares around on a large wall, locality by locality, creating themes for research. A facilitator for each locality described what the wall was 'saying', indicating where interests (red pen) and priorities (blue pen) overlapped. This produced a set of research priorities which were acted on in the following year, led by teams from different geographical areas.

Connected action learning forums for practice manager

In London, up to 20 managers in one PCO meet in a monthly action-learning forum to discuss issues to do with the new GP contract (2004). Each meeting produced three issues or questions which were considered important for others to consider. The issues arising from the group were sent to a bi-monthly meeting attended by practice manager leaders from other PCOs. This group made sense of these in the light of what was happening in other areas and made suggestions for policy makers.

Annals of Family Medicine

The *Annals of Family Medicine* (a US-based international journal for general practice/family medicine; www.annfammed.org) invited e-discussions from diverse constituencies potentially affected by published articles. In a facility called TRACK, new ideas generated from these were fed back into the journal at a later stage, facilitating further developments.

Things you can do to build infrastructures for ongoing learning and change

Create coalitions for ongoing political support

Without ongoing political support from all parts of the system you will be unable to follow through collaborative projects (you will have undoubtedly learnt this during your career so far!). In particular, a network cuts across traditional power relationships, and some will find this threatening. Ongoing political support is needed to avoid harmful consequences.

Politics is 'concerned with the acquisition of power or getting one's way' (*Chambers 21st Century Dictionary*). In this context, 'getting your own way' means protection from forces that might personally damage you, but also might damage the infrastructure of facilitation and communication that is the source of ongoing creative inter-organisational interactions. There need to be formal committees that span the collaborating organisations charged with protecting the shared infrastructure. You need their support. You also need the support of those who influence political developments in less formal ways – opinion formers, people operating in the shadow systems, informal leaders. You must know who they are and include them in your conversations, using them to help you make sense of what is happening locally, nationally and internationally.

All your political supporters need easy-to-read literature and timely information about progress if they are to defend you. Keep them in the loop regularly.

Formal committees to oversee collaborative work are not enough. They can steer or supervise inter-organisational facilitators as project officers or consultants, but organisational ownership requires much greater participation. From this comes ownership of the innovations. One way to enhance organisational ownership is to create teams inside each organisation with a remit to work on complementary parts of a shared initiative. This focuses the attention of the organisational management on the success of their own teams, rather than on what the go-betweens can achieve on their own.

Some things to remember.

- Gaining and retaining a sense of ownership may consume a great deal of your energy.
- The individuals and groups that you first think of may not be the best targets for your attention.
- You may have to give people a great deal of personal support to learn basic skills of partnership working.
- You may need to shift focus to fit with changing political priorities.
- You may need to simultaneously target or support several different groups, setting up a dynamic between them to fuel their further involvement.
- You can better identify where to put your energies by drawing influence diagrams and force-field analysis of the whole system of concern (Chapter 14). These help to deduce where the systemic obstacles to change may lie, and help you to recognise where you may need political help.
- You will need to maintain your own database of political contacts and send them updating information and invitations to take part regularly.

Implications for the clinical encounter

Patients often forget to gain a breadth of support for their plans – perhaps from parents, friends and employers. You can remind them.

Implications for running organisations and crafting policy

Teams inside your organisation need formal and informal support to collaborate with teams from others.

Implications for yourself

You need the right breadth of formal and informal political support, and aim not to draw too much responsibility onto yourself.

Build system maps and timetables

When people can visualise a whole system they can see how to engage with it. System maps and timetables help this. There are multiple overlapping systems that do not necessarily connect. For example, it is common in the NHS for there to be several unreliable and unconnected systems that document childhood immunisation.

You can draw a system map (Chapter 14) to show how different things affect each other. This may reveal 'disconnects' in the system. For example, people in different parts of the system may use different codes to record the same thing.

System maps can help you feel confident in many complex situations – knowing the array of educational courses or self-help groups, for example. You can help a patient to see the multiple inter-connections in their own body by a drawing that displays how various things connect.

When people start to rely on systems for the first time they have to let go of their previous habit of direct personal control. This may give them an uncomfortable feeling that everything is out of control. People used to dominating may forget their promise to adhere to the agreed system and instead try to regain direct control. Less dominant people may fail to point out problems with a system through being unused to take responsibility. These can prevent a systems approach even being tried. You must see this as a normal response that needs patience and persistence to overcome.

To an extent you can ease the discomfort of these people through small projects that produce quick wins. For example, you can draw a flow diagram of referral to a new clinic and use it to analyse ways to improve its efficiency. Similarly, you can provide a clearly visible timeline of a project which helps people to see that things are going according to plan.

You can also bring to people's attention system maps and timetables that already exist but are not recognised as such – care pathways, lists of hospital waiting times, information in a practice brochure. Encouraging people to use them, update them and make them more visible increases their recognition of their value.

When feedback is reviewed about the performance of systems regularly people come to trust and rely on them. With training they can apply the idea in all aspects of their lives.

Implications for the clinical encounter

The way that problems are presented to you by patients often raises expectations of multiple single diagnoses. By drawing a map of how different things connect, you can help them to see how multiple things influence their health all the time. They can see that posture contributes to back pain and debt contributes to depression.

Implications for running organisations and crafting policy

Organisations need system maps and timetables that are easy to retrieve, understand and review. These are needed for staff and patients to understand services and development opportunities.

Implications for yourself

Systems maps and timetables will help you to bear in mind people you need to keep in touch with at various stages of a project. They will help you to recognise where your progress might be obstructed and where support may be needed. Being skilled at creating and reviewing maps and timetables keeps you on top of things and ahead of trouble.

Connect 'nodes' in a system

Nodes are places where different systems connect. At nodes participants learn about each other, gaining windows into quite different worlds of understanding. They are the means of connecting networks of networks.

Examples of nodes are away-days, coffee breaks, social occasions, cross-portfolio meetings, cross-organisational planning groups, conferences and international partnerships for research. In each of these the potential exists for exploring complementary understandings of things that interest you.

Shared need and shared interests can be identified at nodes, and these can be used to form project groups and shared leadership. They pave the way for whole-system learning and innovation. Nodes can be embedded in organisational life, such as team meetings, or developed for whole-system research.[3,4]

Nodes offer particular opportunities for sharing and accessing knowledge, building relationships and getting a better sense of the whole health care endeavour. They need to be facilitated as learning spaces where participants enjoy learning from and with each other. Here, they can meet others, exchange views, form alliances and create projects together. When they are comfortable, reflective and welcoming places they encourage this. When they feel unfriendly and blaming they produce a stifling atmosphere which inhibits creative inter-action.

Clear and thoughtful outputs from learning at nodes are needed to avoid 'noise'. Unfocused, unthoughtful ideas merely frustrate people unless there is an agreed person or group to quickly work further on them so they become more intelligible.

The more connections there are into a node the more important become the signposts that help participants to navigate and participate effectively within them. These include briefing summaries, maps, timetables, descriptions of corporate priorities, aims of a meeting and minutes of the previous ones, and the roles and interests of participants.

Implications for the clinical encounter

The consultation can be seen as a node where patients recognise and reflect on the cluster of things which affect their health. Sequential consultations are connected nodes, helping the patient and you to gain an increasingly rich picture of their situation.

Implications for running organisations and crafting policy

An organisation will have large numbers of places where people habitually congregate. These can be facilitated as nodes where people reflect on the relevance of their work to other places. Ways to use them creatively may be as simple as keeping a list of plans or times of meetings on a wall.

Implications for yourself

You can turn your regular meetings into nodes by ensuring that the right people attend them and they are adequately briefed. This makes your programmes of work connect better, and minimises time-wasting misunderstandings. You need to become skilled at facilitating these meetings in a way that enhances creativity and commitment.

Use backwards mapping to develop strategy

The word *strategy* comes from warfare. It is everything a general does to get the right troops to the right place, with the right equipment, to do the things that achieve goals. Strategy is a complex and multi-faceted plan in which the order of things matters a great deal. If the guns arrive without bullets or soldiers without food, the plan is a failure.

Leaders need strategies that make things happen in the right order. There is no point in the data you need for an annual report arriving after the report has been published. Getting a series of different things delivered on time requires a sequence of co-ordinated activities made easier by an exercise in 'backwards mapping'.[5]

Backwards mapping starts with a clear description of what is wanted at the most peripheral or distant point in the organisation. The strategist works backwards from this to identify what is needed at various stages beforehand. This produces a plan that can be visualised on a timeline. Doing the exercise well gives you confidence that the timeline will bring everything together at the right time.

This approach quickly demonstrates that many things need to come together at the same time and in the same place. These may come from different places – perhaps different disciplines, different parts of a building or from different organisations. For example, if you want receptionists to provide reliable information about the organisation, they need to know staff movements. One step back from this you need all staff to provide up-to-date information about their movements.

Backwards mapping not only helps to achieve a certain goal, it also helps you to identify a set of places where different paths can usefully cross. These are nodes. By standing back and considering the potential value of a node you may find other things which can usefully come together there; for example, you may recognise that the person who holds the list of people's availabilities should also hold the timetable of meetings, annual leave and social events.

Backwards mapping can also help you to cascade information through nodes. Getting the order of cascade right is important if those charged with minding a node are to amalgamate data in time to help the team to make decisions. For example, when writing an annual report there needs to be synchrony between computer downloads, planning meetings and feedback from project leaders.

The same principle of working backwards can help produce personal career and learning plans. They help to plan educational events and manage projects. In each case you: identify what needs to happen, and when; deduce what needs to be in place one step before this; identify the various things needed to bring this about; and so on. Use a big piece of paper and leave it on the wall.

Implications for the clinical encounter

You can help a patient to plan improvement of their own health by mapping backwards from various goals, identifying a set of practical steps.

Implications for running organisations and crafting policy

Organisations can use backwards mapping and sets of co-ordinated timelines to show when information needs to be transferred from one department to another. This displays to everyone how different projects are relevant to each other, and to the development of the whole organisation.

Implications for yourself

The backwards mapping technique helps to plan any situation, from a dinner party to long-term career plans. It will help you to juggle different portfolios effectively.

Exercises

Use the 'Things you can do to build infrastructures for ongoing learning and change'

Read each of the four 'Things you can do . . .' above and decide which is most relevant to your present needs. Write your personal response to this. Include the ideas it brings up for you and what you can practically do. Then do it and reflect on what you have learnt. Make it into an essay to put into your portfolio of learning.

Make a complex power analysis

Consider a system that you want to change about which you feel you know a great deal. Referring to Chapter 14, draw a complex power analysis about this. Reflect on this analysis with a trusted team and discuss the combination of points at which you think your efforts could have most impact. Identify one of these points and do a force-field analysis of this part. In what ways does this help you to decide where to apply your energies, and what coalitions are needed to support long-term sustainability?

Devise a system map

Draw a diagram of one of your organisational systems (Chapter 14). Write in words a description of the same system. Consider in what different ways these two methods of describing a system are useful. How can you use such diagrams and descriptions to make your everyday work more enjoyable?

Create a node

Identify in your organisation different but related streams of work. Invite people from these work streams to meet to reflect on how their work affects others and things they can do to enhance the whole health care effort. Consider whether ongoing meetings of this group can usefully act as a node for the organisation, and what kind of leadership will maximise its potential.

An exercise in backwards mapping

Choose something that you have to lead. It can be an annual report, a personal goal, the completion of a project, or an educational session. On a large piece of paper write down what you need to achieve at that point. Then work backwards to reveal the sequence of things that need to be in place beforehand to achieve this. Stand back and look at this to see if it looks achievable.

Revisit your case study

Re-read your plans about how to overcome your defensive feelings and to support your project teams. Reflect first on how this chapter affirms what you were already planning. Reflect on what new insights the chapter has given you about an effective approach. In particular:

- Is it your previous experience that when people change from direct control to rely on systems they often feel uncomfortable? Did you plan enough of the right kind of personal and political support to follow through?
- Is it your experience that system maps and timetables help people to trust a systems approach? Did you include these things in your plan? Does your plan have clear times for review? Will you be producing a set of timelines to monitor progress? Where will they be on display, and will this be enough for those who need to be able to see them?
- Did you make it clear to the leaders of the project teams that they will be expected to learn from the other groups, and adapt their plans accordingly?
- Did you include in your plans a 'backward mapping' analysis to ensure you have identified the best places for pathways to cross?

References

1 Graver LD, Springett J, Sands R and Reason P (1997) *Evaluation of the Local Multi-disciplinary Facilitation Teams.* John Moores University Project Report, Liverpool.
2 Thomas P and Graver LD (1997) The Liverpool intervention to promote teamwork in general practice: an action research approach. In: P Pearson and J Spencer (eds) *Promoting Teamwork in Primary Care – A Research Based Approach.* Arnold, London.
3 Thomas P, Oni L, Alli M, St Hilaire J, Smith A, Leavey C et al. (2005) Antenatal screening for haemoglobinopathies in primary care – a whole system participatory action research project. *British Journal of General Practice.* 55: 424–8.
4 Thomas P, McDonnell J, McCulloch J, While A, Bosanquet N and Ferlie E. Increasing capacity for innovation in large bureaucratic primary care organizations – a whole system participatory action research project. *Annals of Family Medicine.* 3: 312–7.
5 Elmore RF (1979) Backward mapping: implementation research and policy decisions. *Political Science Quarterly.* 94: 601–16.

Chapter 7

Having the right information at the right time

Summary

Leaders need to see a full picture to decide what are the best next steps.
They need quick access to different kinds of knowledge, and meaningfully
relate this to the evolving stories.

External to your area of influence you need to map the sources of
information and secure permission to access them. Within your area of
influence you can construct relational databases to make one form of data
relevant to others.

By anticipating what analyses will be needed, and when, you can pre-
programme your databases to build the reports in real time.

A case study produces a rich picture by gaining multiple different insights
into the same situation. A combination of quantitative, qualitative and
participatory approaches is ideal. When an organisation operates as a
'learning organisation' or 'learning community' it becomes skilled at
making sense of different kinds of information as a whole. When team
members themselves make sense of data this motivates them to think and
act creatively.

Regularly dipping in and out of your sources of information will help you
to become familiar with their potential. You can use reports of projects to
build organisational memory.

Leaders need to see a full picture to decide which are the best next steps. You
particularly need to see a full picture when there is sudden unexpected change,
such as a local crisis, a new government directive or the loss of a key person. Even
for routine planning you need to feel reassured that day-to-day work remains
relevant to the bigger evolving story.

You need quick access to different kinds of knowledge – policy changes, data
from local projects, newly published research and soundings about how different
people estimate your work.

You can often predict what information will be needed, and even when. By
analysing when information will be needed, you can set up systems to access it at
those points.

External to your area of influence you need to map sources of information and
secure permission to access them. You need to know how data are presented in
order to gather them in a compatible format.

Within your area of influence you can construct inter-related databases to amalgamate complementary information. Databases are commonly designed for one purpose only – perhaps to monitor projects or to track payments.

You can produce complex analyses and different reports from an inter-related database. By having anticipated which analyses will be useful, you can even programme the database to produce them in real time, showing you the shape of a final report long before it is needed.

Doing this, however, requires initial planning which incorporates the views of your team members. Brainstorming, team debates and cross-organisational agreements are needed to make different information useful as a whole. Reflecting as a team on the value of the reports produced by the database will help to improve the databases year on year. Failure to do this may result in team members deciding not to input certain data or inadvertently losing the connections between one part of the database and others.

Using information gathered for one purpose for another purpose is cheap and can enhance efforts for integration. It requires co-ordination. Consider the following.

- Using learning needs identified in personal appraisal to inform educational provision. A summary of learning needs from personal appraisals can be amalgamated and given to education providers. This can help to devise education programmes.
- Meeting the learning needs of individuals when addressing organisational needs. A summary of the learning needs of individuals within an organisation can be compared with the development needs of the organisation. This can reveal a group of people who could address their learning needs and develop aspects of the organisation at the same time.
- Creating combined research and audit projects. A quantitative research project may expose that there is poor impact of an innovation, but be blind to the reasons for this. A simultaneous qualitative audit might reveal the reasons simply by asking the people involved.
- Using project monitoring to show changing patterns of engagement. A database to monitor the progress of research and audit projects could also record which disciplines led the enquiries. This will reveal the changing profile of local engagement.
- 'Real' financial planning. A database to record payments will give a misleading understanding if it fails to consider financial commitments of the next financial year.

In this chapter I explore ways to use information imaginatively to help you and your teams see bigger, richer, more connected and reliable pictures.

Choose your case study: anticipating what knowledge you will need, and when

An introduction to this section can be found at the start of Part II.

Choose whichever of the following case studies is most like your own situation. These are the same cases described in the previous chapters so you may like to look back to see how the story has unfolded so far. Write down your initial ideas about how to manage the situation. Review these at the end of the chapter to see if your ideas have changed.

Developing a general practice

Things settled down in the practice. You had to calm a few people who were feeling unsettled. You had to intervene in one group to help resolve a clash of personalities and you asked one member of another group to hand their role over to someone else because they could not attend the meetings. But the three project teams produced good work. The diabetes and clinical governance teams worked together, since improved care for diabetes had become a priority for everyone. They met regularly with the PCO diabetes group.

With help from the external facilitator, the 'system transformation group' designed an ambitious format for the second all-team meeting, which included a highly effective role-play. Each system redesign team presented their plans to a panel made up of other team members. They were invited to bid for an imaginary sum of money to move forwards their suggested pilot project. The panel scored each team bid according to its feasibility, the strength of the argument about its value and its intended synchrony with other things that were going on. Then, in a plenary session, participants debated what action should be taken.

The event was energising and fun. Evaluation showed that participants learnt a great deal. New ideas emerged. Three pilot projects were unanimously endorsed and the groups leading them gained a spontaneous round of applause. You felt that everyone was now hooked on the process. You can already see the project teams starting to integrate their work.

Now you face the difficulty of proving that this can work in the long term. You are worried that your teams may not have the skills or stamina to follow through. You are also unsure what data you will need to demonstrate its long-term sustainability. You ask yourself: What evidence is needed? How are you to going to co-ordinate data gathering? How can each project be best evaluated in its own terms, and also all three evaluated 'as a whole' to build a sophisticated understanding of the value of your work?

Write down how you will anticipate what evidence you will need, and when.

Developing a community hospital

Things settled down. Everyone other than you seems to have forgotten the behind-the-scenes objections that so unsettled you. The project teams include some very experienced people who quickly produced impressive discussion documents about the options for the community hospital. The three groups met to compare progress on four occasions and by the time of the second whole-system event had well-rehearsed ideas. The political acceptability of these was checked informally through senior managers. There seemed to be increasing concordance between what the project teams and what the directors of the PCO were thinking.

The PCO Board discussed the ideas before the second whole-system event and agreed that the hospital should remain as community-focused as possible, support community services and intermediate care, and provide a bridge between the work of primary and secondary care. The Board was not in favour of keeping open the operating theatre. The Director of Public Health commissioned an options appraisal from an external group.

The build-up to the second whole-system event was fraught with political tension. The Board was rumoured to: support closure of the operating theatre and one of the wards, and support a terminal care/respite centre adjacent to a proposed new-build centre for elderly care; downgrade the accident and emergency unit and provide an intermediate care facility for patients with diabetics and elderly people with mental illness; enhance the community services by the attachment of social workers and community psychiatric nurses; develop a centre for community support to be managed by a consortium of community groups to provide information about local services, including welfare benefits, legal and debt advice, and opportunities for self-help. Gossip was rife. The newspapers were full of off-the-record opinions. But no one knew for certain.

The second whole-system event went very well. The three project teams presented confident and coherent plans. They included baseline data about diabetes care from GP computers, which had been gathered by the PCO diabetes group. The effect of cross-team planning was evident since the three plans fitted well together. Rumours about the views of the Board were largely correct and the chief executive followed the three presentations with a formal presentation of proposals from the Board. The absence of dissenting voices demonstrated the effect of behind-the-scenes negotiations. The rest of the day revolved around adding detail to the broadly agreed plans. The conference accepted your suggestion to adopt a 'real-time strategic change model' (Chapter 16) for future developments. You can already see the project teams starting to integrate their work.

You now have a need to prove it can work in the long term. The political argument has been won – for a while. But intermediate care for diabetes as you have led it to become must prove itself, or else within a few years new political battles will threaten a swing in other directions.

Write down how you will anticipate what evidence you will need, and when.

Developing primary care in localities

Slowly, your three project teams start to produce things. The topics of diabetes and mental health captured many people's interest. The diabetes group acted faster than the others and you used this as an example to spur on the others. One group had a spontaneous change in membership when things failed to progress. You held two more quarterly locality events and the three teams slowly gained prominence at these. You were able to support individual members to think through their personal development needs.

The teams were given impetus when plans for the local community hospital also prioritised diabetes, mental health and the elderly. Soon your teams were leading workshops at the local community hospital where they met with consultants and community nurses. Increasing contact between the hospital and the locality groups resulted in agreement to pilot a model of intermediate care for diabetes, a centre for the elderly at the hospital and the piloting of a new approach to mental health (as yet unspecified). Secondary care consultants from the local teaching hospital became enthusiastic about more of this work being done locally. GPs became enthusiastic about local access to specialist services. Community nurses became enthusiastic about better local connections. You can already see the project teams starting to integrate their work.

You now have a need to prove it can work in the long term. The locality development agenda was set for a while. There was energy for change and leaders were emerging. But the new arrangements had to demonstrate their worth. Unless local collaboration for services proves itself to be more cost-effective than existing arrangements, and the new complex sets of relationships can be consolidated, within a few years new political battles will threaten a swing in different directions.

Write down how you will anticipate what evidence you will need, and when.

An image of multiple complementary insights: the case study

A case study produces a rich picture by gaining multiple different insights into the same situation. It builds up a rich understanding of the whole story.

A case study is a research or audit method that:

> investigates a contemporary phenomenon within its real-life context, especially when the boundaries between phenomenon and context are not clearly evident . . . you would use the case study method because you deliberately want to cover contextual conditions.[1]

it is:

> not either a data collection tactic or merely a design feature alone but a comprehensive research strategy . . . Case studies can be based on any mix of quantitative and qualitative evidence. In addition, case studies need not always include direct, detailed observations as a source of evidence.[1]

Quantitative, qualitative and participatory approaches to enquiry contribute different insights into a case study (Chapter 11). A 'quantitative enquiry' counts named things and later compares figures, perhaps using statistics – different rates of immunisation is an example. A 'qualitative enquiry' avoids advance decisions about what exactly is to be discovered and asks open questions to explore new interpretations that are later clustered into themes through a 'grounded theory' approach – asking women why they do or don't have cervical smears is an example. 'Participatory enquiry' helps people with real-life experience to contribute to the enquiry at every stage, generating knowledge through sharing their complementary insights – practice teams and patients together investigating fair and sensitive ways of offering appointments is an example.

A case study ideally uses all three approaches – quantitative, qualitative and participatory. It can provide a breadth of insight to help you feel confident about 'holding the story'. This will help you to engage with others when arguing your perspective.

Pause

Are you able to describe your work as a case study?

A model that frames a breadth of understanding

This model takes the form of a matrix (Figure 7.1). It works well when laminated as a large sheet (60 × 85 cm). Participants in a workshop place stick sticky squares in different boxes to build up lists for each category.

Across the top of the matrix are headings: Experience; Attitudes; Skills; Knowledge; and Tangible outcomes. These reflect the different domains of learning that are needed for the success of a proposed innovation. For example, in the case of the elderly, an innovation might include practitioners having: the experience of listening to the life stories of an elderly person; valuing the contribution older people make to a community; skills of identifying depression and dementia in elders; knowledge of voluntary centres; and providing information and day centres.

Down the side of the matrix are different headings to indicate places where learning and change are needed: Individual change; Organisational change; Inter-organisational or system change; and Wider change. For example, in the case of the elderly, an innovation might include improved understanding by elders of how the system works; better access in general practice for people with mobility problems; better communication between social workers, occupational therapists and general practice; and adequate pensions.

Each participant in a small group (typically four to six people) writes their ideas on sticky squares. One at a time they place them on the matrix in the place that seems most appropriate, explaining to the group why they think it belongs there. If the group thinks an idea belongs in more than one place they write it more than once.

When everyone has finished, the whole group discusses the whole matrix, noting particularly where there are few or no comments. They check boxes where there are no sticky squares because, here, changes may be needed that no one has yet recognised to be important.

At a plenary session each group summarises the overall shape of its matrix with a brief resumé of the ideas. This usually reveals that different groups have emphasised different things, thus reinforcing the need to create a set of complementary strategies for change, and to evaluate a complementary set of changes. The ideas on the matrices can then be written up as data that both informs the debate about health need and describes sets of data needed to measure success. A summary can also contribute to the debate in the partner agencies about policy for elderly care.

Examples of complementary insights that help make sense of an evolving story

Liverpool Health Promotion Clinic Attendance Project

A participatory action research project entitled the 'Liverpool Health Promotion Clinic Attendance Project' helped practice teams to reflect in workshops on the reasons why women did or did not attend health promotion clinics. Two practices from deprived areas took part. Each had a branch surgery in a relatively affluent area. Thus, there were four sites served by two sets of GPs. A co-ordinated

What changes will be seen?

Where change will be seen	Experience includes all experiences, irrespective of whether people learn from them, e.g. visiting other organisations	Attitudes includes values and beliefs – the ways in which people think and judge others	Skills includes the things people can practically do, e.g. listen	Knowledge includes the things people know, both as facts and deeper understandings	Tangible outcomes includes organisational and service developments such as team meetings and new clinics
Individual change change in individual people					
Organisational change change in individual organisations					
Inter-organisational or system change including communication systems and networks					
Wider change not in the local system					

Figure 7.1 An evaluation matrix.

sequence of workshops between the practice teams led to an increasingly sophisticated understanding of the issues as perceived by the practice teams. The researcher then interviewed a selection of women and fed back to the teams what they had said.[2,3] The recognition that the women were saying the same things as the practice teams, but with different emphasis, caused a magical moment of empowerment for the practice teams. They enthusiastically adopted the changes suggested by the research.

Liverpool Medical Audit Advisory Group

The Liverpool Medical Audit Advisory Group (MAAG) developed sustained support for reflective multi-disciplinary audit throughout the city. The group coined the phrase 'audits of quantity, quality and consensus' to imply the complementary value of exploratory qualitative audits and consensus-creating audits, as well as traditional quantitative audits. When new resources for health promotion were made available, the MAAG, working with the Family Health Services Authority, agreed that a combination of all three audits was a marker of quality. MAAG facilitated a series of four two-hour workshops in six locations in the city, cascading learning from each stage to subsequent workshops, both at the meetings and by post.[4] This resulted in the formation of multi-disciplinary practice teams which debated what different audits would give optimal insight to their work. Sixty-seven per cent of all practices attended the workshops (74/110) and more than 80% of practices produced multi-disciplinary strategies that included these three different approaches.

Whole-system participatory action research 1

A 'whole-system participatory action research' project explored the potential for screening pregnant women for haemoglobinopathies in general practice instead of in hospital.[5] Quantitative data about dates of screening were complemented with qualitative data from key informants. At whole-system events, stakeholders from different parts of the system debated the meaning of these data in the light of their own experiences. This revealed that general practice screening was able to reduce the gestational age of screening, but the changes in working practice of everyone involved made this an unrealistic innovation.

Whole-system participatory action research 2

A different whole-system participatory action research project used comparative case studies, qualitative interviews and surveys to explore what features of a primary health care bureaucracy facilitated learning and innovation.[6] At annual whole-system conferences stakeholders reflected on the meaning of data. Over three years the insights became increasingly sophisticated, identifying five features which supported learning and innovation and three that caused low morale.

Research network

A research network recorded for each project the name of the lead researcher, date of completion and the publications that followed. By also gathering the designations of other research team members and local presentations made by the teams a picture of the changing pattern of research participation and local impact was gained.

General practice system

A general practice system for repeat prescriptions was devised so that administration staff could print prescriptions without patients being seen by a doctor. This meant that drugs given only in consultations were invisible in that part of the computer system. This could potentially result in an incorrect description of the total list of drugs that a patient was taking. By including all medications that a patient was taking regularly, but coding them differently, it was possible for administration staff to print them and also to identify all medications that a patient used regularly.

Family practices in the USA

Family practices in the USA are required to analyse feedback forms from patients about quality of care. By coding responses by age, sex, ethnicity and geography, and by comparing them with the numbers sent out it was possible to gain a fuller understanding of how well the practice served different population sub-groups.

General practices in the UK

General practices in the UK record aspects of care on their computer systems for financial payments and these are analysed by the PCO. In north-west London there are plans to set up the PCO databases in such a way as to permit local interrogation for local research and audit, as well as for reimbursement purposes. This will allow some practices to undertake collaborative research and others to provide a morbidity surveillance mechanism.

Things you can do to have the right information at the right time

Devise a personal knowledge retrieval system

There will be times when you need to pull together information from a variety of places at the same time. Commonly, intelligence arrives late or cannot be accessed, or you are too overwhelmed by other things to get it. For knowledge to be there when you need it, you need to plan.

You need to know what kind of knowledge might help you. To do this write down: what reports and papers you may need to write; what interests you have; what things you may want to prove; and what things you may need to defend against. For each of these, identify what knowledge you might need and where you might get it.

You can consider journals, libraries and web resources as well as data you generate yourself. People you know may have useful ideas about what sources are useful and accessible.

By writing into your schedule regular times to dip in and out of these resources you will become familiar with what they can offer. By regularly practising retrieval of information, you can become skilled at getting it quickly. Pressure of time will tempt you to always use the same sources, so at least some 'butterfly' reading is useful. Try auditing what you read and in what ways it helps you. This is especially useful when writing papers or applying for funds, and when undertaking projects because these reveal resources of practical use. Your thinking and actions about these can all contribute to your professional portfolio of learning that builds the story of your own development.

You can develop your own library, at home or at work. This can include reports generated by your organisation about audits, projects and significant events. These can document the development of your organisation, and build the organisational memory.

Retrieving knowledge easily from your own sources requires that you are familiar with your own categorisation systems. If these are the same categories used by your teams and other groups you will be able to retrieve things for each other.

Your categorisation systems are easier to remember when they mirror your everyday work. Try displaying your system of computer folders as a picture on the wall. This will help you see how you can design it to be more closely related to your day-to-day concerns. You can make your different systems mirror each other – computer folder skeleton, system for storing papers, books in your own library, projects completed. Standing back from time to time to examine the categories you have constructed helps you to see their coherence as a whole, and whether they fit the ways other people categorise things. The more things mirror each other the more you will feel that you know your way around. This will give you confidence in your ability to use them effectively.

Implications for the clinical encounter

You can search for information with a patient in a consultation. This requires you to be skilled at navigating your favourite databases for disease diagnosis and management, service options and self-help.

Implications for running organisations and crafting policy

Lists of useful databases and training in knowledge management can be shared throughout an area. Libraries can be accessed and local data amalgamated. You can provide dedicated space for staff to surf the internet, try out software for research and understand the systems.

Implications for yourself

You need a reliable list of knowledge sources that make sense to you. You need to be skilled at using them, and have well-rehearsed ways of filing and retrieving knowledge.

Design multi-purpose databases

By knowing what reports you want to write, at what times, you can design databases that produce these with minimal extra effort. Conversely, if you try to produce a report without this initial planning you will find yourself casting around for information that is difficult to access and in incompatible formats.

You can program databases to amalgamate data in a compatible way. For example, a database may be needed to record which audits are being undertaken. By adding to the data-gathering sheets the designation and home organisation of project team members you can also produce reports on the changing pattern of engagement in audit by discipline and location. If your database also records the research projects being undertaken you can show the changing pattern of engagement in both audit and research, revealing to you something of the organisational capacity to undertake rigorous enquiries.

Information is often held in different places in incompatible formats. It is sometimes possible to align the dates, boundaries and denominators in these different data sets to display comparable data. Sometimes it helps merely to know where these different databases are and secure permission to use them.

Some databases are already designed to combine different data. GP computer systems are an example of such an integrated package. Gaining agreement from different general practices to gather data in a co-ordinated way can release the power of these systems. It requires standardised ways to input and export data. For example, collaborators need to agree whether to amalgamate data by calendar year or by financial year. Calendar year data has advantages because it is easier to present year-on-year changes; and it allows time in the spring to amalgamate data from different sources for annual reports in April.

Clear times for people to review amalgamated data helps data-management systems to remain sensitive to the emerging needs of the organisation and sector. Timely feedback of amalgamated data helps people to see its value. Leaders make sure that feedback happens at the best times, and key informants reflect on how the system should be changed for the following time.

Teams with responsibilities to think through comparable data-gathering have useful experience with which to devise knowledge management systems for PCOs and strategic health authority areas.

Implications for the clinical encounter

The patient record in a GP computer is a multi-purpose database. You can use this in your consultations to show patients how different information about them is helpful. Similarly, patient-held records can help different clinicians to record comparable data.

Implications for running organisations and crafting policy

The PCO needs to produce many different reports for different purposes. These can often be anticipated in advance, and databases pre-programmed to produce the reports you want when you want them. These can be synchronised across a sector to show changing patterns throughout large areas.

Implications for yourself

Careful thought in advance about what indicators will help you to demonstrate your impact may permit you to modify existing databases to generate this evidence.

Coordinate the timelines of multiple related projects

There will be times when you need to pull together intelligence from multiple projects at the same time. You will also want intelligence from one project to inform others at the appropriate time. This is unlikely to happen easily unless the leaders of those projects understand why this matters and reliably produce data at the agreed times.

The technique of 'backwards mapping', described in Chapter 6, helps to identify what timelines are realistic. It was originally developed as a management tool to permit 'street-level discretion' (providing management support to people at street level or on the periphery 'elbow room' to be creative).[7] It identifies what needs to be done at the most peripheral point and works backwards. This contrasts with the more common approach to management that starts from the needs of the top and works downwards.

Different people can see how their work fits into a bigger scheme of things by a display of connected timelines. These show how different programmes of work overlap with others. These can be displayed together on the wall as multi-coloured charts, each with different stages appropriate to that project. Nodes – places where different people and outputs come together – can be clearly marked. An example is the annual report, but there may be other places where work from one work-stream needs to input to others, or cross-pollination of ideas between project teams is desirable.

Individuals may not be experienced at producing realistic timelines. They may need options to change their plans in the light of unexpected circumstances. They will need feedback of amalgamated information to show that their contribution has been useful.

Leaders of different work-streams can develop their own graphic display of connected time-lines of their own projects. This will help them to devise plans that are connected, and notice at an early stage when things are falling behind. Teams can use backwards mapping to plan co-ordinated gathering of information. For example, one person could review peer-reviewed journals and another health service guidelines, both providing information in time for other teams members to gather data from the field.

Implications for the clinical encounter

You can negotiate with patients who have multiple problems a co-ordinated review of several things at the same time. For example, repeat medication, screening blood tests and physical examination may all be needed. Agreeing with a patient an appropriate frequency of these and the rationale of co-ordinating them helps you and them. This approach is time-efficient because several things are done at the same time. It is empowering because patients gain better control of their personal plans. It is a way of increasing your practice targets by motivating patients to get things done on time.

Implications for running organisations and crafting policy

Organisations can use the technique of connected timelines as a way to encourage cross-portfolio working and keep track of a variety of projects.

Implications for yourself

Personal coordinated timelines will help you to meet your various goals and feel in control of things even when they seem chaotic.

Nurture the stewards of organisational memory

Organisational memory can be lost by the departure of one or two people. Organisational memory reminds people why things are done in a certain way. It accesses resources. It helps to value infrastructure and culture that has been taken for granted. It is necessary for organisational learning.

Stewards of organisational memory often have things to offer other than knowledge about the past. They often contributed to the creation of the organisation and carry respect and authority. They may know how to solve problems by accessing the right people at the right time. Knowing who they are helps to use them wisely, and keep them on your side. You need to be clear about what memory is needed and who is guarding it.

Consider memory to be the strings holding balloons of knowledge. The person holding the strings of those balloons is a steward. The organisation keeps a map of the domains of organisational knowledge (balloons) and ensures that there are enough stewards to retain them all in an effective way. When a balloon string is under threat, the organisation needs to act. Balloons, in this sense, can be organisational portfolios. The leader of a portfolio is responsible for ensuring that various aspects of the past are remembered.

You can map the domains of organisational memory, and identify who are their stewards (Chapter 14). You need to bring to their attention, and the attention of others, that you value this. You can demonstrate that you value them by using their knowledge in various ways and feeding back what happened as a result of their involvement.

You can ask all those who lead audits, projects and significant events to produce their reports in ways that will document the development of the organisation, building the organisational memory through a series of project reports to be held in your library.

You need to consider succession planning for the stewards. You can extend the group of people knowledgeable about their domains by building teams around them. You can make sure that systems and contacts in this domain are written down in ways which can contribute to a written organisational memory.

Implications for the clinical encounter

It is common for people to forget about their family and cultural roots. From time to time you may need to help patients to remember where they can access information about these at a later date. Does someone hold a family tree? Where are wills and the deeds to the house? Who are the people with whom they have fallen out, and might they at some future date wish to rekindle a relationship? Who would they like invited to their funeral?

Implications for running organisations and crafting policy

Leaders of different portfolios may need to be guided to understand and value the historical context of the work they are leading. They may need introductions to, and friendships with, those who remember another time, who can help them to retain infrastructure and value hard-won principles. They may need help with succession planning.

Implications for yourself

You need to be clear about what areas of expertise you have, and which of your colleagues is keeping track of things that are important to you. Inside your teams you can reach agreements about what each expects from others and what you are prepared to provide, so you become clearer about the organisational roles you hold.

Exercises

Use the 'Things you can do to have the right information at the right time'

Read each of the four 'Things you can do . . .' above and decide which is most relevant to your present needs. Write your personal response to this. Include the ideas it brings up for you and what you can do practically. Then do it and reflect on what you have learnt. Make it into an essay to put into your portfolio of learning.

Devise your own knowledge retrieval system

Brainstorm (Chapter 14) the different domains of knowledge that you need and what journals, books, reports and other resources are relevant to these. Then write where you can access them, and allocate regular time to explore them.

Devise a multi-purpose database

Consider a database over which you have some control. Write down what its main purposes are. Brainstorm (Chapter 14) a list of other purposes that it might serve. From this list identify a small number of indicators that could easily be generated from the database at little extra effort. Consider the advantages and disadvantages of monitoring these.

Devise a set of coordinated timelines

Make a list of different things you need to coordinate. They can be personal or work-related. Identify when you want them to connect. Write a set of co-ordinated timelines. Stand back and see if this shows you how they usefully connect.

Identifying stewards of organisational memory

Ask who knows most about the history of the organisation. Seek out and interview these people with the intention of understanding better why the organisation is as it is, and which various individuals are stewards of different aspects of it past and its external relationships. Consider what areas of knowledge may be under threat and how you will continue to access organisational memory.

Revisit your case study

Re-read your plans about how to get the right information at the right time. Reflect first on how this chapter affirms what you were already planning. Reflect on what new insights the chapter has given you about an effective approach. In particular:

- Did you identify databases within the organisation or network that you can use? Did your plan involve your three project teams themselves identifying what data they need in order to evaluate their progress?
- Did you identify a set of external sources of data for yourself and for your project teams? Did this include qualitative as well as quantitative data, and have you designed a way for local people to take part in making sense of these data as a whole? Did your plan include team support to access information? Are you building a list of useful information sources and making them easy for people to access?
- Did you devise with each team a timeline that was feasible, and which would deliver results in time for the next feedback session? Did this cross with the timelines of the other groups at the best times before the next event, so they could start to develop their ideas in synchrony with the other teams?
- Have you started to explore the domains of knowledge held by the people in the organisation? Have you considered ways to highlight important things that are taken for granted? Did your plans include discussing with stewards of the organisations' memory their preparedness to access knowledge and people on behalf of others?

References

1 Yin RK (1994) *Case Study Research*. Sage, Thousand Oaks, CA.
2 Leavey C and Thomas P (1995) *Advancing Health Promotion, Research and Policy*. Institute for Health, John Moores University, Liverpool.
3 Leavey C (2000) *Why do women not attend for cervical smear appointments?* (dissertation). Centre for Health, Healing and Human Development, John Moores University, Liverpool.
4 Thomas P (1994) *Report: The Liverpool Primary Health Care Facilitation Project 1989–1994*. Liverpool Family Health Services Authority, Liverpool.
5 Thomas P, Oni L, Alli M, St Hilaire J, Smith A, Leavey C *et al.* (2005) Antenatal screening for haemoglobinopathies in primary care – a whole system participatory action research project. *British Journal of General Practice*. **55**: 424–8.
6 Thomas P, McDonnell J, McCulloch J, While A, Bosanquet N and Ferlie E (2005) Increasing capacity for innovation in large bureaucratic primary care organizations – a whole system participatory action research project. *Annals of Family Medicine*. **3**: 312–17.
7 Elmore RF (1979) Backward mapping: implementation research and policy decisions. *Political Science Quarterly*. **94**: 601–16.

Chapter 8

Looking after yourself

Summary

Leaders make the most of the present moment. You only have the present moment to do anything about anything.

A common threat to balance is when engaging with those who see things differently from you. This may be at a meeting when explaining the point of view of the people who look to you for leadership. It may be within conflict, perhaps when people are attacking you. In these situations it may help to remind yourself that you can learn from these people. If feeling defensive remind yourself that you have covered to the best of your ability the areas described in the previous chapters of Part II: you know the story (Chapter 4); you are facilitating learning about its evolution (Chapter 5); you are building infrastructure for ongoing learning and change (Chapter 6); and you have the information you need to back up your claims (Chapter 7). If you have done these, your challenge is not to bow to pressure from others, but to speak your truth as well as you can, and to learn from the situation. To do this you need to keep yourself alive in the present.

Meaning lies in making past memories and future hopes coherent to each other, and to the evolving story. This meaning is woven in the present. Being preoccupied with regrets or fears prevents you from doing this. Many techniques help us to remain centred in the present moment, acknowledging multiple tensions without being damaged by them. You need to find techniques that suit you.

There is often a slim margin between getting it right and getting it badly wrong. Anxiety about every step can lead you to forget to look after yourself, or those on whom you rely. Rigorous attention to planning and review is more likely to get things right.

No one source of knowledge will reliably tell you what to do. Instinct, logic and advice of trusted friends and objective informants are all helpful ways to interpret evidence. You need to keep up the activities you know are good for you, and to trust what you could see on clearer days.

'Projection' is the phenomenon of attributing success and failures to others when they should be better attributed to you. Certain techniques can identify projections and attribute them more appropriately.

A blaming or dismissive mindset will not recognise the good that exists in difficult situations and, consequently, will be weak at finding imaginative ways forward. Appreciative mindsets are more effective.

Members of high-performing teams can run off the ball, carrying the trust of other team members that they are making this move for the good of the whole team. To take part in this creative play, teams must first become

> rehearsed in more ordinary team skills of passing the ball back and forwards to each other.

Leaders make the most of the present moment. Each person has only this moment to do anything about anything. Into the present you carry past memories and future hopes. Meaning lies in making these coherent to each other, and to the evolving story. Being preoccupied with regrets or fears prevents you from doing this. It prevents you from being alert to the extraordinary potential of the present moment.

Being alert in the moment requires being clear-sighted within multiple uncertainties and changing agendas. At least a tightrope walker knows where the other end of the rope is tied. As a leader you may often feel that you are walking along multiple ropes, the other ends of which lie in some unknown future place. There is often a slim margin between getting it right and getting it badly wrong. Anxiety about every step can lead you to forget to look after yourself, or those on whom you rely. Or you might give way to fatalism and forget the power you have to make a difference. Both are likely to inhibit your potential.

A common threat to balance is when engaging with those who see things differently from you. This may be at a meeting when explaining the point of view of the people who look to you for leadership. It may be within conflict, perhaps when people are attacking you. In these situations it may help to remind yourself that you can learn from these people. If feeling defensive remind yourself that you have covered to the best of your ability the areas described in the previous chapters of Part II: you know the story (Chapter 4); you are facilitating learning about its evolution (Chapter 5); you are building infrastructure for ongoing learning and change (Chapter 6); and you have the information you need to back up your claims (Chapter 7). If you have done these, your challenge is not to bow to pressure from others, but to speak your truth as well as you can, and to learn from the situation. To do this you need to keep yourself alive in the present.

No one source of knowledge will reliably tell you what to do. Instinct, logic and advice of trusted friends are all useful. Keeping up the activities you know keep you balanced is helpful. You should trust what you could see on clearer days.

You can make moments stretch when you give people a sense that you are there fully for them. Conversely, when you seem distracted you waste time, disconnecting from people and missing things of importance. Being alive in the moment means 'listening to the whispers' – seeing important things that may not actually be pointed out or put into words. This helps to make leaps of imagination and see windows of opportunity. It helps to quickly get past 'noise' to see the things that really matter.

Seeing advantages for creative action in the moment does not mean that plans should change from one moment to another. Plans should be carefully, painstakingly, worked out to the best of your ability and with participation of your teams. Other people rely on them. They should not be discarded lightly. Nevertheless, when key assumptions inside them are no longer true a rethink is needed.

You will need to speak in the language of whatever group you are working with. You may have feet in many camps. You may be at the centre of cultural conflicts. You may find that everyone wants a part of you when things are going well and everyone wants to blame you when things go badly. Your greatest successes may permit others to do things for themselves that leave you out of the credits. This success can threaten your own understanding of who you are and where you belong.

A disciplined personal care programme and breadth of techniques to deal with stress can help you to remain buoyant in the high seas.

Your case study revisited: attaining personal balance

An introduction to this section can be found at the start of Part II.

You have reached a point where some order has emerged in the situation you are leading. It has taken a long time of what seems to you like constant misunderstandings and conflict, but now there is a sense that things are under control. Your multi-disciplinary events and pilot projects have produced outputs of value. There is a buzz of energy about the place that was not there before. The support from your organisational partners is holding and your teams are showing increasing able leadership skills and integrated activities. You expect the third whole-system event to approve policy that will sustain progress. You intend to stand down after this event, or at least renegotiate your role.

You feel tired and a bit unappreciated. Few people seem to have noticed how much you have carried on your shoulders. Your quiet, behind-the-scenes problem solving, personal support of staff, protecting them from 'above' have been a large part of this success. But your work has been invisible to many important people, and dissenting voices say that you have been too slow to deliver and are a 'soft touch'. Some people have demonstrated a malicious determination to harm you.

You also feel confused inside. You have become used to seeing things from many different perspectives and have lost the sense of who you are. You sometimes feel that you have feet in every camp but no camp of your own. You do not even know where to turn to for help. You find the theory of this multi-perspective world overly challenging. You find the techniques to help different people to understand each other test your skills to the limit. It feels that you are always operating at the edge of chaos, and committing to more tasks that you can complete. You long for a simpler world.

Write a plan to manage these tensions inside yourself.

Images that hold creative tensions

In this chapter the image box is empty. It is for you to fill it with images that speak to you. Try a selection of images and bring them to mind in different circumstances. You will know that they work when they help you to remain balanced in difficult situations.

The image does not have to be a picture. It is anything that you can bring to mind in order to calm inner anxiety and be grounded in the present. It can be a reminder about something you know about yourself – 'you are a good person'. It can be the memory of a hero – 'be like Gandhi'. It can be a physical movement – a smile. It can be a stirring piece of music or a favourite scent.

Try different images in different contexts. When in conflict you may find helpful the image of a martial arts expert, throwing someone with their own weight; or the image of a reed bending in the wind; or the serene Buddhist calm in the midst of noise. What helps you to overcome the sensation of tiredness – the face of a smiling child, the image of skiing down a mountain? Athletes, dancers, orators, flowers, music, smells, friends, heroes – all can provide images that will remind you what to do to acknowledge tensions and hold them, changing them into a force for good.

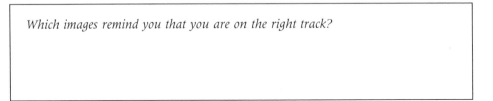

Which images remind you that you are on the right track?

A model of self-development: a flotilla of boats

Figure 8.1 shows several boats, loosely connected by ropes. The flotilla is you – your whole life story. Each individual boat is a sub-plot, a significant strand of your identity. This image is intended to remind you that there are many strands to your life story, and moving one strand forwards can leave others adrift.

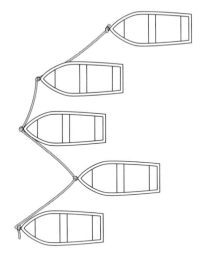

Figure 8.1 A model of self-development: a flotilla of boats.

For example, you may forget how important music or dance once were to you, as you divert time to your professional development or to family affairs. In time this neglect will show itself and you may experience a sense of general dissatisfaction, or resentment of the constraints that your own success has caused.

You have responsibility to yourself to bring into view from time to time the various 'boats' – interests, needs or sub-plots that define the whole of you. Name them. Write them down. Make resolutions to tend them. Make yourself a set of timelines to move them forward and make them more relevant to each other – pulling better together.

Examples of things that facilitate balance

Being balanced requires a degree of strength in all dimensions of health – physical, mental, social and spiritual. You may find it helpful at pivotal moments in your life to reflect on what you need in each of these domains for the challenges ahead, and to devise a plan to achieve them.

The question you face is whether these things are in balance appropriate to your challenges. An athlete performing in the Olympics has different need for health than the same athlete when playing ball with her daughter.

Health can be improved by doing everyday things differently. You can take the stairs rather than a lift, centre yourself between appointments and use images and breathing to calm inner voices of doubt. You can train all your senses to be alert in the moment.

Techniques that help us to be alive in the moment are to be found in the literature of stress management, career and life management, self-development, spirituality and meditation. Different people prefer a different combination of approaches.

Here are some examples.

- Chambers and Davies write about managing stress.[1] They encourage you to keep a diary to make sense of the various things that cause you stress at work. Focusing on one page a day, you are encouraged to score your mood and make associations with things that affect it. Techniques for posture, time management and team support are all covered.
- Career and life management consultants present tried and tested exercises to help you analyse and develop your personal skills, aptitudes and ambitions.[2]
- 'New age' practitioners provide powerful exercises in visualisation to see your present situation with new eyes.[3,4]
- Religious and spiritual groups have a variety of approaches to being still in the moment.

These resources all encourage breathing control, meditation, visualisation, general fitness and 'hearing the whispers'. The image of 'narrative unity', described in Chapter 12, reminds us that our choices in each moment are important and personal. Meaning lies in making the past and future meaningful to each other in the present moment. Stress is not intrinsically wrong – it is a challenge for growth.

Things you can do to remain buoyant in the moment

Use images and phrases that keep you alive in the present

With the best will in the world the pressures of daily life will at times force you to feel that you have 'lost the plot'. This can be a prolonged 'dark night of the soul', or a temporary distraction. It can even be your dominant habit. You can reduce the damaging effects of this by using images and phrases that remind you of times when you could see things in a more optimistic way. The aim is to keep you balanced and alive.

A common threat to balance is when engaging with those who see things differently from you, especially when they are critical of you. In these situations it may help to remind yourself that you can learn from them. It may be better to understand and help them than to assert your authority or prove them wrong. You should anticipate these moments of misunderstanding and have to hand the evidence to set right incorrect facts.

You may need to rise above the stress of the moment that will lead you to say or do things you will regret. Images that are meaningful to you may help you to keep alive in the present. From your past you may find helpful pictures, completed work or friends. From your future you may find useful the plans that remind you of your intended trajectory.

Your aim is to keep focused on what the people around you are saying, both in words and what they really mean. You need to keep at bay the internal voices that cause self-doubt. You need to be able to feel the tensions around you and inside you, and rise above these to reach out to understand the others.

A disciplined programme of exercises can increase your skills at doing this. You may notice no difference there and then, but like a trained athlete, when the pressure is on you will show your strength.

You need to be aware of the extraordinary power of the mind. Faith really can move mountains! As Henry Ford said, 'If you think you can or you think you can't, you're probably right.' Mental models are powerful determinates of success and failure. You can learn to switch them on and off, and use different ones in different contexts. Like an actor on a stage you can move between different ways of thinking and acting. It takes practice to do this convincingly, but skills gained can help you in every aspect of your life. Try exercises of visualisation to mentally rehearse how you will do something (Chapter 17).

A *simple rule* is an easy-to-remember directive that can switch on a mental model. 'Fight to the death' is a simple rule that relates to the mental model of 'I will overcome my adversaries'. 'The customer is always right' is a simple rule that relates to the mental model of 'the best way to gain customers is to keep them happy'. It is time well spent to examine what mental models you want, and what simple rules will switch them on.

Implications for the clinical encounter

Patients commonly feel lost and isolated. You can help them to find images and words that keep them going while they grope for coherence.

Implications for running organisations and crafting policy

Policy must help staff to manage stress and remain alert in the midst of change and conflict. Senior management support and good team-working are essential to develop mutually affirming images.

Implications for personal balance

You will need to discover those images and phrases that keep you alive in the moment. You will need to practise them and be reflective about the effect they have on you. If you are not able to be alive, happy and effective in the middle of the multiple forces which threaten to knock you off balance, you may need to reconsider your plan.

Deal with projection

'Projection' is a common phenomenon. It means attributing success and failures, strengths and weaknesses to others when they would be more accurately attributed to ourselves. It arises from the mental models that govern what we are able to see. However, we become confused and think we are seeing others when we are detecting our own preferred way of looking.

We are particularly likely to be blind to our harmful projections at times of stress.

Projection of previous unresolved hurts seems particularly common, perhaps because this is painful to look at honestly. Hurts work away in our deeper psyche to produce negative ideas about ourselves. These ideas bubble to the surface and project onto others. This act of blaming other people diverts attention away from looking at the actual origins of these harmful ideas – which lie inside the accuser.

Knowing about projection helps us to recognise that when we see something in someone else that we do not like, we may be seeing a part of ourselves that needs attention. Similarly, when we see something we admire in someone else we may also be seeing a part of our own self about which we are insufficiently aware.

This awareness reminds us to be cautious about accepting the labelling of others – good or bad. It reminds us to give people space to give their own account of themselves. It reminds us to do the same things with ourselves, better appreciating our own ideas, motivations and potential, rather than accepting uncritically the flattery and criticism of others.

It helps us to avoid behaving like victims. It reminds us to remain self-critical but also self-protecting. We can say to critics: 'I know you don't see things the way I do but I am prepared to listen you. Convince me that I am wrong and I shall change – but until that happens I have no realistic option but to retain my views'.

It reminds us to keep in close contact with those who understand our way of seeing things but at the same time not to isolate ourselves from other world views. This will help us to keep things in perspective when feeling accused or rejected, and also in the midst of adulation and success.

It reminds us that our friends and colleagues may struggle with similar issues. We can strengthen them by checking out with them from time to time how we honestly perceive each other. They especially need us when they are feeling weak.

Implications for the clinical encounter

Open questions and active listening can help to reduce projection of the feelings of the clinician onto patients. What patients say, and don't say but signal in other ways, needs to be treated seriously. Sometimes it needs to be challenged gently. Trusted relationships help to do this. You also need ways to deal with the hurt they may project onto you.

Implications for running organisations and crafting policy

Organisations, and society generally, need to nurture a leadership style that recognises projection and has positive ways to deal with it. This involves careful listening to all sides of a dispute and not rushing in to judge on the basis of untested ideas.

Implications for yourself

You need to understand your own potential to project your own feelings onto others. If you have strong feelings inside, whether good or bad, calming techniques can help prevent you projecting them onto others. You can consider them to be signals of your own development needs. When someone else projects feelings onto you, you similarly need techniques to avoid being overly affected by them.

Convert bad into good

> 'Things are so bad, they can only get better,' said Eyore . . . 'Oh no,'
> said Pooh, 'things can *always* get worse.'

The best way to make sure that things get worse is to focus on the bad and ignore the good things that are always to be found. However, completely ignoring what is going wrong is also unwise. A balanced position is, first, to be clear about the nature of the good and bad, then to build on the good in a way that solves the problems of the bad. In time the bad comes to be seen as the thing that stimulated the new good growth. With hindsight it was 'a Good Thing'.

A blaming or dismissive mindset will not recognise the good that exists in difficult situations and, consequently, will be weak at finding imaginative ways forwards. When something seems wrong it may well indicate that something needs to be done (it may not) – but it does not necessarily tell you what to do. Often, something that seems to be wrong does not need to be removed, but complemented by other things. Often, the thing that is obstructing progress is out of your immediate vision and you need to look wider – the problem may be you!

Appreciating others is a powerful way of getting the best out of them. Appreciating yourself is a powerful way of getting the best out of you. You can only build from a positive. It is difficult to build a positive equal relationship from a blaming mindset. Appreciative enquiry is an excellent method to identify positive things from which to build.[5]

Adopting an appreciative style does not mean that you avoid highlighting and confronting things that are wrong. However, it does require that criticism be complemented with practical, positive suggestions about how to do things better. It means constantly reaching out to others. It means giving constructive feedback to others which helps them to see how to build from things they are doing right rather than feeling blamed for things they are doing wrong.

The more you practise appreciative approaches the more you will recognise how frightened people can be when out of their comfort zones. This makes them less able to learn and do what most needs to be done.

You can empower people to look at these difficult things by helping them to put temporary boundaries around situations, which enable them to work through realistic but ambitious plans. You can do this by seeing change as 'incremental revolution', as described in Chapter 13. You can do it through play, which is an effective way of creating safe boundaries – children do it all the time. The Mary Poppins image from Chapter 4 encourages you to regularly use the approach in real-life as well as in training courses.

People will often gain confidence from your positive intentions whether or not you get the words right. When you catch the wrong note, a swift apology and humour can often turn things in a positive direction. Success comes from developing a large numbers of different ways of turning 'no' into 'yes'.

Implications for the clinical encounter

Empowering patients to take control of their health is helped by an appreciative mindset which recognises and builds from the good and puts the bad in context. Humour, identification and slight irreverence are useful to help people to identify positive things they can build from.

Implications for running organisations and crafting policy

Organisations need to encourage ongoing reflection on both good and bad, using both to steer in positive directions. A blaming and unappreciative culture produces defensive and unhappy staff. Well-timed and constructive feedback is a powerful motivator.

Implications for yourself

As a facilitator of change you will need to be skilled at seeing hope in the most difficult situations. It takes patience, discipline and experience to remain calm, attentive and appreciative, especially when people are blaming you.

Run off the ball

If a creative football player runs off the ball he creates openings. He finds space. He changes the state of play. This is a successful tactic only when other team members recognise his skill, are rehearsed in such movements and trust his integrity to play for the whole game rather than his own glory.

This skill is needed in all high-performance teams if they are to release the potential of the moment. Your teams will only be able to do this if they are rehearsed in ordinary set pieces. Flashes of genius require good grounding in the basic principles of ordinary team life.

You can help team members to run off the ball by devising an atmosphere of trust and mutual understanding. This requires that all team members become prepared to give things a go and be unafraid to fall. They must know from experience that when they cannot quite pull things off, the team will support them, laugh with them and help them to learn how to pull it off next time. Shared projects are a good way to learn and practise these team skills.

To develop your own abilities to 'run off the ball' you will need to belong to high performing teams. You need to keep up to date with how team members are growing – or else you may expect too little, or the wrong kind of thing.

Implications for the clinical encounter

When you have a trusted relationship with a patient you have room for lateral thinking. This can often unblock obstacles and expose good ways forwards. This 'running off the ball' might come from referring back to something sensitive that they previously confided, or jokingly rehearsing alternative, crazy options, or voicing something you are sensing that is unspoken. Continuity of care, team-working and family-oriented records help this because they provide hooks into different aspects of someone's life.

Implications for running organisations and crafting policy

Organisations need to be able to think 'out of the box' if they are to take imaginative leaps forward that will meet future needs. Policy must encourage individuals and groups to challenge the status quo, in a constructive and appreciative way.

Implications for yourself

You can develop these 'Mary Poppins' skills by facilitating group games, and getting others to enjoy taking part in potentially risky adventures of discovery.

Exercises

Use the 'Things you can do to remain buoyant in the moment'

Read each of the four 'Things to do . . .' above and decide which is most relevant to your present needs. Write your personal response to this. Include the ideas it brings up for you and what you can do practically. Then do it and reflect on what you have learnt. Make it into an essay to put into your portfolio of learning.

Identify the domains of your own health

Draw a set of boats and label each with a different thing that matters a lot to you – things that are important aspects of your identity. Continue until you can think of no more areas (boats). Score each from –5 to +5 about your satisfaction with the present situation.

   In red pen, draw lines to connect those boats which strongly need each other to move forwards. In blue pen, draw lines to connect those boats where advance in one is likely to push the other back. Redraw the whole picture on a grid marked –5 to +5, rearranging the boats on the appropriate grid marking. Stand back and reflect on what you see in the overall pattern. In green pen, draw tentative connections between boats that you had not previously considered, and which might improve the overall pattern. Also in green, indicate the boats you intend to move forwards and backwards in the next period. Write conclusions for action. Write the date on the picture and keep it safe so you can review it another time.

Explore the extent to which you appreciate yourself and others

Make a list of people who are important to you for personal and professional reasons. Go through each name and ask yourself what things you can do that will make them feel appreciated by you. When did you last do this? Revisit the same list and ask what things they can do to make you feel appreciated. When did they last do this? Ask yourself if this points to anything you need to develop in your relationships.

Explore projection in yourself and others

Consider something you like in someone. Write down as clearly as you can what is this trait; then ask yourself if this is a trait that you also have or would like to develop. Score out of 10 the degree to which you think this trait describes you, and them.

Consider something you dislike in someone. Write down as clearly as you can what is this trait; then ask yourself if this is a trait that you also have. Score out of 10 the degree to which you think this trait describes you, and them.

Consider something positive and something negative that has been said of you by others that struck you forcibly. Write down as clearly as you can what this trait is, then ask yourself if this is a trait that *they* also have. Score out of 10 the degree to which you think this trait describes you, and them.

Share your writings with a trusted friend, perhaps asking them also to score you. Compare the scores and discuss the implications.

Convert bad into good

Consider something of your past that you think of as 'bad'. Using a 'life-line' technique (Chapter 14) draw from this the good things and the bad things that happened as a result. Use different-coloured pens to distinguish them. Note if both good and bad can come from the bad things. Second, write your ideas in a third colour about how the good things could address some of the bad things. Write a plan to act on this insight. If you cannot find optimistic ways forward, consider gaining advice from someone skilled at helping people to resolve past hurts.

Identify potential for 'running off the ball' in your teams

Consider one team, of which you are a member, that you consider to be high-performing, and another that is performing at a lower level. Identify a time when you or someone else did something unexpected for the sake of the team, expecting the rest of the team to respond in a creative and appreciative way. To what extent did this happen? How did this make you feel? Analyse what you need to do in each of these teams to develop them.

Devise images and phrases to keep you alive in the present

Re-read the section 'Images that hold creative tensions'. Write a series of images/phrases/simple rules that you think might help you. Put them somewhere where you can see them regularly – in your pocket or on your wall, for example. Reflect on the effect they have on you when you use them.

Revisit your case study

Re-read your plans about how you are going to manage the tensions you experience. Reflect first on how this chapter affirms what you were already planning. Reflect on what new insights the chapter has given you about an effective approach. In particular:

- Do you recognise the phenomenon of projection? Does this idea help you to re-interpret any accusations or praise that has been targeted at you? Does it help you to re-interpret any accusations or praise that you have made of others?

- Are you adequately appreciative of others? Are you adequately appreciative of those closest to you? Are you adequately appreciative of yourself? Do you regularly give others constructive feedback, and demand it of them? Are you able to identify hopeful things in damaging situations – or do you tend towards self-pity and blame? How are you going to gain better balance about these things?
- Are your teams high-performing? Are they rehearsed at passing the ball skilfully to each other? Do they recognise 'running off the ball'. Do you have their trust so that when you run off the ball your teams recognise this as a team tactic rather than a run for personal glory? How are you going to improve these team skills?
- Name your various teams. What purposes do they fulfil for you? Are you nurturing them enough? What teams are missing and how are you going to bring them into being?

References

1 Chambers R and Davies M (1999) *What Stress in Primary Care! The once in a lifetime programme that will help you to control stress in your practice.* Royal College of General Practitioners, London.
2 Hopson B and Scally M (1999) *Build Your Own Rainbow – A Workbook for Career and Life Management.* Management Books 2000 Ltd, Chalford.
3 Edwards G (1995) *Living Magically – A New Vision of Reality.* Piatkus, London.
4 Edwards G (1996) *Stepping into the Magic – A New Approach to Everyday Life.* Piatkus, London.
5 Whitney D and Trosten-Bloom A (2003) *The Power of Appreciative Inquiry.* Berrett-Koehler, San Francisco, CA.

Part III

Theories of integration

In Part III, I explore incompatibilities in the mental models commonly held by people about primary health care, knowledge, health and change. I suggest ways to overcome these incompatibilities. In particular, I explore how movement between linear and systems thinking helps genuine integration.

I am mindful of the statutory role to develop integrated primary care of UK primary care organisations (PCOs) (termed 'primary care trusts; PCTs, in England). These network-like organisations serve populations that range in size from fewer than 100 000 to 250 000, and hold the contracts of all general practices in this area. In many places (for example, London) the boundaries are co-terminus with the local authorities, in order to facilitate partnership working.
PCO/PCTs have three roles:

- to promote and protect the health of the public
- to provide community services, such as district or community nursing
- to commission hospital care for the local population.

These roles are being reviewed and the provider function may become separated from PCOs that will retain a commissioning role. This would require a new home for community services and for leadership for whole-system development.

They incorporate public health, including responsibilities for research and development, and health promotion.

When developing strategy for health, PCO/PCTs will encounter among their diverse stakeholders incompatible ways of thinking in three different areas.

- Different people think differently about the nature of knowledge – a theory of knowledge able to integrate different assumptions about reality is needed. This requires broad agreement that knowledge generated in one context may not be relevant in others.
- Different people think differently about the nature of health – a definition of health able to integrate different aspects of health is needed. This requires recognising that people need to make sense of their discrete health problems in the context of their whole life stories.
- Different people think differently about the nature of change – a multi-layered, participatory and co-evolving understanding of change is needed. This requires broad agreement to develop a synchrony of effort between those who lead short-term incremental change and those who lead long-term whole-system transformation.

Linear and systems thinking are both needed

Below I summarise the chapters of Part III. In each chapter I emphasise that 'systems thinking' and 'linear thinking' need to happen at the same time. Each sees very different things within a whole picture. Each is insufficient on its own.

Linear thinking dominates theories of science, health and change. It is the idea that the world is 'naturally' ordered into discrete unchanging particles which affect each other in direct and predictable ways, like hitting a billiard ball. In the 'real world' multiple billiard balls interact, and each ball is itself undergoing ongoing change, making the billiard ball image somewhat limited.

Linear thinking on its own isolates factors that are really inter-connected, and simplifies things that are really complex. It leads to a static view of a world that is really moving. It leads to ideas about management and change which stifle innovation and promote defensive behaviour.

Linear thinking promotes a black and white, cut and dried, view of the world. At its worst linear thinking sees a person as a set of diagnoses, learning as a passive accumulation of facts, change as the result of force, and enquiry as a way to reinforce the status quo.

Linear thinking leads to the understanding that health is a 'state' that can be objectively measured and meaningfully compared with the health of others. This provides a useful snapshot of the state of society as a whole, but it does not show what health means to individual people, nor what to do when many factors are affecting health at the same time.

Nevertheless, linear thinking is both unavoidable and desirable. It predicts behaviour in simple situations. It provides a focus for purposeful action. It gives a sense of control – and from this the confidence to engage further in an uncertain world.

Systems thinking does not see discrete controllable particles. It sees dynamic interactions between related things. There are many schools of thought. I refer to Bertalanffy, Capra, Checkland, Maturana and Varela in Chapter 1. As a sole approach it is limited – it promotes ambitious vision without practical application. It needs to be complemented by focused linear thinking and targeted action appropriate to the needs of the moment.

In the following five chapters I want to examine the relationship between linear and systems thinking. The reason is that I perceive a popular desire to keep them apart, or to assume that one or other is more important. I wish to persuade you that they are equal but different – and whatever people say, in reality they do a bit of both. Leadership for integrated primary health care must be skilled at moving between the two.

Common sense tells us that people switch backwards and forwards between these mental models. When that bus is bearing down on you, you do not pause to discuss the transport system – you jump out of the way. When you are tending a garden you put the flowers that like the sun on the wall that faces the sun. In Chapter 1 I suggest that 'common sense' is a powerful and profound form of mental juggling that moves between linear and systems thinking.

However, academics and health practitioners alike commonly argue that we must think in one way or another to be 'rigorous'. Moving between them loses objective validation that discerns 'good' from 'bad'. I prefer to argue that academics and practitioners have yet to agree how to rigorously move between the two, and validate knowledge that is generated from different theories of knowledge.[1]

I hope to demonstrate that both linear and systems thinking are always relevant, although we may need to emphasise one or other for specific reasons. Second, I wish to argue that practice, enquiry and integrated health care all require both. Third, I wish to argue that all situations need a mechanism to permit dynamic movement between these two mindsets that allows those involved to make sense of the unfolding story.

A similar argument unfolds in each chapter.

- Comprehensive primary health care (concerned with all aspects of health) and selective primary health care (concerned with targeted interventions) are complementary. The mechanism to decide how much of each is appropriate at different stages is a dynamic multi-disciplinary 'learning community'.[2]
- General practitioners (GPs) must treat seriously the presenting complaint of a patient, and at the same time help them to feel a more empowered and whole person. The mechanism to do both is a dynamic, interactive 'narrative-based' approach to consulting.[3]
- Quantitative and qualitative approaches to enquiry see different and complementary things within a moving picture. The mechanism to crystallise[4] meaning from these different insights is a dynamic 'participatory and action-oriented approach' to enquiry.[5]
- Health involves reducing diseases and also developing the whole person. The mechanism to make these meaningful to each other is a dynamic process of self-reflection to create a coherent 'narrative unity'.[6]
- Leading change for integrated health care requires a sustainable strategy for whole-system evolution as well as discrete inducements for small steps. The mechanism to achieve these short- and long-term successes is an ongoing spiral of whole-system learning and change, inside which complementary 'incremental revolutions'[7] motivate further progress.

The models and theories of all of these already exist. Many people are already leading this. If you have read this far you are almost certainly one of them. One thing that is lacking is a theory capable of making diverse insights and motivations relevant to each other.

In Chapter 9, I describe the story of 'comprehensive primary health care'. This is a broad understanding of health, agreed in the 1978 WHO Alma Ata Declaration of Health For All (by the year 2000). It expects all aspects of society to contribute, including education, public health and all citizens. Care for the physical functioning of someone's body is only a small part of this broad concept of health. Social care, mental health care, environment health and spiritual care are others, each concerned with different aspects of individual, social or environmental health. Some maintain that comprehensive primary health care has failed, because its target year passed by without sufficient progress, and its vision has been highjacked by a selective, targeted approach that produces linear structures that prevent comprehensive primary health care. However, the values and aims of the more ambitious idea are still very much alive, and there has developed a more realistic understanding of the formidable obstacles to success, and the speed with which they can be overcome. In particular, there is a need to understand what organisational, systemic and individual capacities are needed to support sustainable efforts for simultaneous horizontal and vertical integration. In the UK, moving this forward is the responsibility of those leading practice-based commissioning.

In Chapter 10, I describe the story of 'general practice'. This role originated in specialist medical/surgical care and, for this reason, carries a main aim to diagnose and remove diseases. For many years general practice was left to find its own way, separate from hospital care. This resulted in the idea that GPs help patients and their families with all aspects of their health. It is associated with the term 'primary care', which became prominent in the UK after the 1990 health care reforms, when multi-disciplinary teams became common in general practice. It is the main medical discipline to have regular and ongoing contact with a complete breadth of other disciplines in health care in the community, and, for this reason, could provide a valuable contribution to shared leadership for integrated health and social care, both horizontally and vertically. Overwhelming demands and strong allegiance to linear ideas about science, health and change make this unrealistic without new skills, new kinds of support and new approaches to multi-disciplinary team-working and systems thinking.

In Chapter 11, I challenge the central relevance of traditional (positivist) objective science to the complexities experienced on a daily basis by generalist practice, and to effective learning and change. I suggest that critical theory and constructivism offer equally valid and useful lenses with which to view the world. They relate to qualitative and participatory approaches to enquiry. Second, I argue that knowledge generated by any of these approaches is not truth itself, but a snapshot of more complex and moving stories. To reveal a trustworthy picture, knowledge must make sense of whole stories. A combination of all three approaches to the generation of knowledge is needed, often at the same time.

In Chapter 12, I consider the meaning of health in the light of the limitations of theory as described in Chapter 11. Health is what people need to develop a life story which is meaningful to them. Clearly, diseases affect how a life story will evolve, but they are not the same thing as, and less important than, the story. People seek 'narrative unity' – a meaningful life story. Motivation for change comes from multiple hidden factors within these stories and the web of relationships that forms someone's sense of self. Change that is more than superficial alters this web of relationships and is more likely to be embraced if it enhances the coherence of the story.

In Chapter 13, I consider learning and change in the light of the ideas of the preceding chapters. I draw on the idea of a 'learning organisation' that requires three different types of learning. 'Single-loop learning' involves the accumulation of facts, detection of errors and an approach to change that is incremental. 'Double-loop learning' involves the exploration of new ways of thinking and behaving, and an approach to change that encourages new ways to do things. 'Deutero-learning' involves dynamic interactions between different experiences and ideas to generate new insights about how different things can connect. The concepts of 'learning organisation', 'learning community' and 'incremental revolution' help to develop strategy for ongoing whole-system learning and change. In this chapter I also draw conclusions about the policy implications of the ideas of this book.

References

1 Borkan JM (2004) Mixed methods studies: a foundation for primary care research. *Annals of Family Medicine*. **2**: 4–6.
2 Wenger E (1998) *Communities of Practice – Learning, Meaning, Identity*. Cambridge University Press, Cambridge.
3 Launer J (2002) *Narrative-based Primary Care. A Practical Guide*. Radcliffe Medical Press, Oxford.
4 Janesick VJ (2000) The choreography of qualitative research design. In: N Denzin and Y Lincoln (eds) *Handbook of Qualitative Research*. Sage, Thousand Oaks, CA.
5 Whyte WF (1991) *Participatory Action Research*. Sage, New York, NY.
6 MacIntyre A (2000) *After Virtue*. Duckworth, London.
7 McNulty T and Ferlie E (2002) *Re-engineering Health Care – The Complexities of Organizational Transformation*. Oxford University Press, Oxford.

Chapter 9

What can we learn from 'comprehensive primary health care'?

Summary

In this chapter I describe the story of 'comprehensive primary health care'. This is a broad understanding of health, agreed in the 1978 WHO Alma Ata Declaration of Health For All (by the year 2000). It expects all aspects of society to contribute, including education, public health and all citizens. Care for the physical functioning of someone's body is only a small part of this broad concept of health. Social care, mental health care, environment health and spiritual care are others, each concerned with different aspects of individual, social or environmental health. Some maintain that comprehensive primary health care has failed, because its target year passed by without sufficient progress, and its vision has been highjacked by a selective, targeted approach that produces linear structures that prevent comprehensive primary health care. However, the values and aims of the more ambitious idea are still very much alive, and there has developed a more realistic understanding of the formidable obstacles to success, and the speed with which they can be overcome. In particular, there is a need to understand what organisational, systemic and individual capacities are needed to support sustainable efforts for simultaneous horizontal and vertical integration. In the UK, moving this forward is the responsibility of those leading practice-based commissioning.

What is comprehensive primary health care?

The term 'primary health care' was described at the WHO international conference in Alma Ata in 1978, as a way of thinking about 'health for all'. It recognises the contribution of all citizens and organisations, including education, community development and public health, as well as general medical practice. It goes far beyond what is described as 'primary care' in the UK. Knowledge about its practical implications has largely been generated in the developing world. The idea of primary health care is big enough to include all relevant perspectives for holistic whole-system care. It has room for both medical and non-medical approaches, linear and non-linear understandings of cause and effect, statutory and non-governmental health care provision.

MacDonald describes comprehensive primary health care as:

an approach to the planning of health services . . . much more than an addition to existing health services, much more than medical care. It is a reorientation of all health services towards the health needs of communities, both local and national[1]

He describes the three pillars of primary health care to be 'participation', 'inter-sectoral collaboration' and 'equity'.

Participation

Taking part in initiatives for health improvements and collaborative enquiry develops ownership which makes participants more likely to follow things through. Taking part results in a deeper understanding of what can improve things. Taking part moves forwards participants own understanding in ways that make them increasingly strong advocates of quality health care.

Inter-sectoral collaboration

The aims of 'health for all' touch all aspects of society. Many things affect health. No one agency can meet them all. The environment affects health.[2] Social relationships affect health.[3] Family relations affect health.[4] In order to devise complementary policy and sustainable communications between them, different organisations need to agree their shared purpose, value each other's contributions and develop shared projects.

Equity

The greater the differences in income between rich and poor, the worse is the overall life expectancy of a population.[5] The greater are held the principles of primary health care, including equity, the better is the health of a nation.[6] Gross inequalities between the 'haves' and the 'have-nots' make it more difficult for people to stand side by side, as equal citizens, and work for the system as a whole.

MacDonald is describing both horizontal and vertical integration of health care systems. Horizontally, different disciplines collaborate for health improvement across geographic areas and organisational boundaries. This results in complementary support for individuals with health needs, and opportunities for citizens to contribute to community efforts for health and care. Vertically, care pathways for people with health problems avoid duplication of effort and efficient use of resources.

Achieving simultaneous vertical and horizontal integration requires a complex integrated strategy which allows care pathways and team membership to change in response to the specific context. This sensitivity to local conditions requires local leadership. Like travellers negotiating a complex of railway networks, it requires sets of maps and timetables to help people to navigate the whole system using their own intelligence. Like lost travellers, uncertain of what are their true concerns and options, it requires skilled support to help unpack the breadth of things that are bothering them, and reshape them in ways that help them to make decisions about their future trajectory.

The Liverpool Healthy City 2000 Project

The ambition to realise the ambitions of Alma Ata led to the 'Healthy City 2000' movement. In 1988, Liverpool became one of the first cities dedicated to promoting these ideals.

I took up my post as primary health care facilitator in Liverpool in 1989. This role was originally intended to develop general practice along the lines of the 'Oxford Facilitation Project' (which helped individual practices to solve problems and undertake demonstration projects). However, the authorities agreed to an experiment of a community development model of facilitation – where general practice was the community to be developed. This became an experiment in whole-system learning and change, which I described in Chapter 1.

Our first multi-disciplinary primary care facilitation team formed an immediate alliance with the Healthy City 2000 project team. Together we built a network of multi-disciplinary leadership teams and networks which connected individuals and sectors throughout the city. This helped us all to recognise the inadequacy of existing change theory to describe what we came to call 'pathways to integration'. We considered practical pathways for the issues we encountered – from unemployment to work, from social isolation to community engagement, from inactivity to self-actualisation, and from sickness to robust health. In each situation the winning combination was overt recognition of the length of the journey combined with easy, practical steps. This thinking was significantly at odds with the language of change prevalent at the time, which emphasised single short-term answers to these complex questions.

It helped us to recognise that changes were needed in the mental models of generalist practitioners (medical, nursing, voluntary and welfare rights) towards more complex and long-term journeys. We also recognised a need for change in the thinking of public health to support collaborative projects, community development and systems of support for this more integrated image of society.[7]

In 1993, a Liverpool Health Authority discussion paper acknowledged the broad definition of primary health care required for integrated care:

> Primary health care is the system of support and care provided by everyone in the community for each other which enables them to feel good and achieve everything they are capable of.[8]

This translated into a practical strategy for primary care development:

- co-ordination – ensuring adequate connection of medical provision for care with other provisions
- devolution – producing effective local planning and management
- support for self-help and informal care
- communication, including information about services and interpreting services
- participation in care and planning of different groups, including carers, users and families
- team working
- effective information systems
- adequate quality assurance.

Many of the projects that resulted from this approach are described in Chapter 1 and throughout Part II. But, both the theory and the practice were much harder than they seemed at first sight. As this book shows, I had to go into unfamiliar theoretical territory to make sense of it.

The visionary thinking of Alma Ata is not enough

After the Second World War the same spirit that led to the establishment of the National Health Service (NHS) in the UK led to the inauguration of the World Health Organization (WHO). Fired with vision and representational legitimacy (192 countries, rich and poor, were equal voting members in 2002)[9] the WHO became involved in every part of the globe, articulating ethical policy, setting an agenda for research and development, catalysing change and negotiating partnerships for collaboration.

The spectacularly successful smallpox eradication scheme began in 1967. In 1977, the last case of smallpox was reported in Somalia. Dr Mahler, WHO Director-General, announced the success at a meeting in Kenya in 1978 as 'a triumph of management, not of medicine'. Legend says that he then turned to Donald Henderson, who had directed the smallpox programme, and asked him which was the next disease to be eradicated. Henderson reached for the microphone and said, 'the next disease that needs to be eradicated is bad management.'[10]

The implied criticism of these words was prophetic. In the following year (1978) the WHO international conference of Alma Ata declared 'health for all by the year 2000'. This notion was to develop comprehensive primary health care and redistribution of wealth, both north and south, and within nations. But management theory and practical management experience were not up to something so ambitious. Instead, the year 2000 witnessed increased disparities between rich and poor,[11] claustrophobic globalisation and domination of the WHO agenda by the World Bank, driven by theories of market forces and objective targets.

A pull towards linear thinking

In the late 1970s in the UK, Australia and New Zealand there was a popular perception that the state social sector was out of control. It was deemed to be too expensive and overly dominated by trade unionists and professionals.[12] In the UK these popular concerns swept into power the 1979 Conservative government, led by Margaret Thatcher. A year later Ronald Reagan became the President of the USA. The Thatcher–Reagan alliance led a drive for low state involvement in society, individualism, and the promotion of 'free markets'. This led to the idea of a global market of 'free' trade. The rules of engagement made this an unfair market,[13] but, nevertheless, the idea that individual entrepreneurial activity could succeed captured the imagination of people throughout the globe, encouraging a targeted, competitive mindset. In the UK this pushed things in the opposite direction to integration, for example producing a number of different railway companies whose services did not connect. Thatcher even went as far as to say, 'There is no such thing as society, only the individual and the family.' Developing integrated efforts for health became a low priority.

The Thatcher reforms gave rise to 'New Public Management' (NPM). Writing in 2001, McNulty and Ferlie[12] identified four different NPM types. The earliest, NPM1, made the public sector more 'business-like', which, by the mid-1990s, had evolved into NPM2, in which downsizing, decentralising and quasi-markets were strong features. NPM3 arose from the 1980s literature on 'excellence', including 'soft' management that emphasised human creative potential, charismatic leaders and learning organisations. NPM4 was emerging as they wrote and highlighted the value-base of public sector organisations; it included public/private partnership, a concern with quality (e.g. total quality management; TQM), the language of users rather than customers, elected rather than appointed bodies, and a stress on societal learning.

WHO policy was considerably affected by the drive to targets. In 1980, Walsh and Warren argued that comprehensive primary health care as advocated was not attainable. Instead, there should be 'a selective attack on the most severe health problems . . . directed at preventing or treating those few diseases responsible for the greatest mortality'.[14]

The emphasis on targets was dominant in *Health of the Nation*[15], which heralded the UK government strategy for health care reform throughout the 1990s.

Other agencies, such as UNICEF, agreed. UNICEF identified a set of priorities called GOBI-FF – an acronym for 'Growth monitoring, Oral rehydration, Breastfeeding, Immunisation, Family planning, Food supplements'.[16]

Advocates of comprehensive primary health care were doubtful that this was wise. Selective initiatives such as GOBI produced hierarchical vertical management structures that prevented the development of the horizontal integrating structures needed for comprehensive primary health care.[17] Mahler, the WHO Director-General, expressed disappointment at this unforeseen turnaround.[18]

A pull towards whole-system thinking

Other countries developed a more integrating philosophy. From the point of view of the UK/USA, the Gorbachev reforms of the Soviet Union from 1985, and the fall of the Berlin Wall in 1989, were validations of capitalism, encouraging further application of market theory to international policy. But, from the point of view of continental European countries such as France and Germany, there was an urgent need to deal with two Germanys, and to integrate former Soviet States into a united Europe. They also had practical experience of developing the European Union,[19] and had been influenced by continental hermeneutic philosophy[20] that offered a theory of consensus-creation between people. This produced a tension between the philosophy of heroic, direct action from the UK/USA and the continental European approach which preferred to negotiate an accord between different perspectives. This tension was played out in a dramatic way in their different preferred strategies in the (second) Iraq war.

In other countries, methods to produce participatory approaches to democracy were being tested. In Africa and Asia, models of participatory enquiry within primary health care were developed.[21] The *African National Congress 1994 National Health Plan* in South Africa proposed ambitious plans for participatory primary health care and whole-system transformation. However, mainstreaming these ideas proved difficult, and targeted approaches remained dominant.

How to develop integrated and participatory health care systems in the mainstream was debated in a series of WHO conferences. Conclusions were summarised in the 1996 Ljubljana Charter. This proposed that health care systems should be:

- driven by values of human dignity, equity, solidarity, and professional ethics
- targeted on protecting and promoting health
- centred on people, allowing citizens to influence health services and to take responsibility for their own health
- focused on quality, including cost effectiveness
- based on sustainable finances, to allow universal coverage and equitable access
- oriented towards primary health care.

The European community adopted these principles in 1996.[22]

The language of integration came back into UK and USA politics through the Clinton/Blair language of a 'third way'.[23] This emphasised the need for social as well as individual health, and complementary needs – signalled by the catch-phrase 'rights and responsibilities'. The (New) Labour government of 1997 expressed its intention to create integrated multi-disciplinary primary care: 'the basis for a 10 year programme to improve the NHS . . . [by] a replacement of the internal market by a system of integrated care'.[24]

In 2001 McNulty and Ferlie critiqued the contribution of post-1997 New Labour government to the development of the 'new public management' in the UK. They concluded that despite the use of Giddens' language of the 'third way', and Leadbetter's ideas about 'modernisation' there was little evidence of new models of lateral integration. They concluded that the New Labour approach 'is essentially NPM1 orthodox'. 'Top-down' targeted, linear thinking was as strong as ever in the UK health service. They concluded 'vertically based principles of organizing are likely to remain important and indeed dominant within the NHS and perhaps other UK public services'.

PCOs came later. I describe in Chapter 3 that my reason for being hopeful about PCOs goes beyond their statutory obligation to facilitate integrated health care. To my eyes they are a manageable size, and happening at a time in history when there is better understanding of the principles of integration. Also, they are likely to form coalitions of general practices for 'practice-based commissioning' (devolving commissioning for services to a more local level) and this could facilitate local collaborations between many different stakeholders.

However, as I write in 2005, PCOs are struggling. Overwhelming workload and insufficient experience are preventing efforts for integration. The disbandment of the Modernisation Agency, the failure of the NHS University and threatened further organisational restructuring do not give confidence that a brighter future is over the horizon.

But it is too early to tell. There are clearly people who care deeply that a health service is created where participation, equity and inter-sectoral collaboration are natural everyday preoccupations. The structures exist to develop a systems-aware health service. In all respects conditions are more favourable than those we inherited in Liverpool in 1989. Theory and models of complex inter-organisation change and sustainable development have moved forward in leaps and bounds in the last 16 years; team-working has improved; the language of whole systems and participatory approaches to enquiry has a legitimacy that was just not there only a few years ago. It all hangs in a delicate balance.

A need for combined linear and whole-system thinking

Dr Bruntland, who became WHO Director-General in 1998, acknowledged the need for a combined systems/focused approach to management in her message in the 2000 World Health Report.[25] She wrote:

> One of my prime concerns [when taking up office] was that health systems should become increasingly central to the work of WHO . . . Recommendations should be based on evidence rather than ideology. (p. vii)

The same report attributed the 'failure' of comprehensive primary health care as a mismatch between needs and wants:

> Despite its many virtues, a criticism of this route [comprehensive primary health care] has been that it gave too little attention to people's demand for health care, and instead concentrated almost exclusively on their perceived needs. Systems have foundered when these two concepts did not match, because then the supply of services offered could not possibly align with both. In the past decade or so there has been a gradual shift of vision towards what WHO calls the 'new universalism'. Rather than all possible care for everyone, or only the simplest and most basic care for the poor, this means delivery to all of high-quality essential care. (p. 3)

But this policy to agree a 'bottom line' of care has not done away with the more ambitious idea of complex integration. Xingzhu Liu, in her 2003 review of options for health care systems,[26] identified the lack of mechanisms to shift resources to this end:

> Although there is evidence that allocation of resources to primary and preventative care, which is highly cost effective or even cost saving, will improve allocative efficiency, there seems to be no clear mechanism for achieving the desirable resource shifts. (p. 5)

Her report concludes a number of practical things that can support integration:

- good information systems, and reliable evidence, including applied research and teams of experts (p. 117)
- building capacity for better connections between research and policy change, collaborations between researchers and policy makers, and prioritising diseases/risk factors (p. 118)
- technical support and economic evaluations (p. 119)
- measuring provider performance and toolkits (p. 120).

'Building capacity for better connections' means much more than expert researchers and policy makers. It also means developing organisational and systemic capacity. It means developing systems-aware leaders. It means developing an infrastructure of facilitation and communication to support integrated primary health care.

Primary health care, social cohesion, healthy public policy – and the problem of medicine

Shared leadership and an infrastructure of communication and facilitation for integrated primary health care will clearly also be needed to achieve the United Nations' 'Millenium Development Goals':

- eradicate extreme poverty and hunger
- achieve universal primary education
- promote gender equality and empower women
- reduce child mortality
- improve maternal health
- combat HIV/AIDS, malaria and other diseases
- ensure environmental sustainability
- develop a global partnership for health.

This list reminds us that comprehensive primary health care is not the only need. Also needed are 'social cohesion' to protect and develop local communities and 'healthy public policy' to reduce the social fragmentation that is the experience of so many societies and to promote collaboration for health promotion in its broadest sense.

In March 2005 a background paper for the WHO Commission on Social Determinants of Health (CSDH) provided a frank and articulate account of the twists and turns that have thwarted the aims of Alma Ata and led to 'health strategies that fail to address the social roots of illness and well-being'.[27] The paper reminds the reader of the central relevance of horizontal integration of diverse efforts for health and social care, acknowledged in the 1995 World Summit WHO Position Paper: 'health issues could be most effectively addressed through inter-sectoral collaboration to tackle factors such as poverty, unemployment, gender discrimination and social exclusion'.

First among their eight key strategic questions is:

> How will the CSDH position itself on the Mahler–Grant problem' – between a far-reaching structural critique based on a social justice vision [comprehensive primary health care] and promoting a number of tightly focused interventions that will produce short-term results, but leave the deeper causes of avoidable suffering and health inequities untouched [selective primary health care]?

It states that:

> a significant challenge for social determinants of health and health equity agendas will be bringing the medical establishment on board as a constructive partner . . . [because] physicians have a strong group interest in maintaining their monopoly over authoritative discourse and practice around health

and are:

> reluctant to see control of health issues slip away from them to other sectors and professional constituencies, or to cede to communities the power to set health agendas.

They claim that the fundamental reason for this pattern is economic – doctors make money from curative programmes.

I believe that it is not solely, or even mainly, the medical establishment that is the obstacle but the linear mental model which underpins medical thinking. Sustainable whole-system integration requires the pillars of primary health care – participation, equity and inter-sectoral collaboration. These all require an acceptance that things are equal but different, connected within systems rather than arranged in a hierarchy of importance. The linear and compartmentalised theories of knowledge, health and change that doctors are obliged to use are unable to fully engage with these non-linear and relativistic concepts.

Pointing a way to bridge these linear and systemic worlds is my hope for this book. GPs and family physicians more than any other could become the bridge-makers because they naturally have so many windows into different worlds of understanding.

Implications for primary care organisations

Insights from many countries about how to gain widespread collaboration for health throughout whole communities may help PCOs. Both the practice and the theory are difficult and a concerted effort is needed to better understand them.

Formative and continuing learning of practitioners and managers should include skills to apply the principles agreed in the Ljubljana Charter, including values of equity and human dignity, health protection and promotion, people-centredness, focus on quality and sustainable funding. Chapters 2 and 4 describe an approach to leadership able to facilitate ongoing application of these principles. Chapter 6 describes how to build infrastructures to support this.

Professional groups and academics must explore the interface between linear and systemic thinking to agree a reliable way to make them meaningful to each other.

Leadership should systematically develop the three pillars of primary health care: participation, inter-sectoral collaboration and equity.

Skills of participation can be developed through 'learning spaces', including community-based projects and multi-disciplinary work-based learning (Chapter 5).

Skills of inter-sectoral collaboration can be developed through networks, whole-system events, shared projects and whole-system audit and research (Chapters 6 and 7).

Equity awareness can come from participation in consensus-creation and community projects, using networks to understand different perspectives, and interrogation of data-sets at a local level (Chapters 5, 6 and 7).

Brenda Foran from the University of Western Sydney Australia provided material and references for this chapter. My thanks to her.

References

1 Macdonald JJ (1992) *Primary Health care – Medicine in its Place.* Earthscan Publications, London.

2 Hume-Hall R (1990) *Health and Global Environment.* Polity Press, Cambridge.

3 House J, Landis KR and Umberson D (1988) Social relationships and health. *Science.* **241:** 540–5.

4 Huygen F (1990) *Family Medicine – the Medical Life History of Families.* Royal College of General Practitioners, Exeter.

5 Wilkinson R (1992) Income distribution and life expectancy. *BMJ.* **51:** 478–85.

6 Starfield B (2000) New paradigms for quality in primary care. *British Journal of General Practice.* **51:** 303–9.

7 Ashton J and Seymour H (1988) *The New Public Health.* Open University Press, Buckingham.

8 Liverpool Healthy City 2000 Project (1993) *Primary Health Care in Liverpool, A Discussion Paper – Towards a Model of Primary Health Care Based on the Principles of Health for All.* Liverpool.

9 Yamey G (2002) WHO in 2002: why does the world still need WHO? BMJ. **325:** 1294–8.

10 World Health Organization (2005) *The World Health Organization Smallpox Eradication Programme.* WHO, Geneva.

11 Werner D and Sanders D (1997) *Questioning the solution: the politics of primary health care and child survival with an in-depth critique of oral rehydration therapy.* Healthwrights, Palo Alto, CA.

12 McNulty T and Ferlie E (2002) *Re-engineering Health Care – the Complexities of Organizational Transformation.* Oxford University Press, Oxford.

13 Klein N (2002) *Fences and Windows. Dispatches from the Front Line of the Globalization Debate.* Flamingo, London.

14 Walsh J and Warren K (1980) Selective primary care: an interim strategy for disease control in developing countries. *Social Science & Medicine.* **14:** 145–63.

15 NHS Executive (1991) *Health of the Nation – A Consultative Document.* NHS Executive, London.

16 Mull J (1990) The primary health care dialectic: history, rhetoric, and reality. In: J Coreil and J Mull (eds) *Anthropology and Primary Health Care.* Westview Press, San Fransisco, CA.

17 Newell K (1988) Selective primary health care: the counter revolution. *Social Science & Medicine.* **26:** 903–6.

18 Walt G (1993) WHO under stress: implications for health policy. *Health Policy.* **24:** 125–44.

19 Dedman MJ (1996) *The Origins and Development of the European Union 1945–1995.* Routledge, London.

20 Wulff H, Pederson A and Rosenburg R (1990) *Philosophy of Medicine – An Introduction.* Blackwell, Oxford.

21 De Koning K, Martin M, Tandon R, Maguire P, Meulenberg-Buskens I, Tolley EE *et al.* (1996) *Participatory Research in Health: issues and experiences.* Zed Books Ltd, Johannesburg.

22 Starfield B (1998) *Primary Care – Balancing Health Needs, Services and Technology.* Oxford University Press, Oxford.

23 Giddens A (1998) *The Third Way.* Polity Press, Malden.

24 Department of Health. *The New NHS, Modern, Dependable.* HMSO, London.

25 World Health Organization (2000) *The World Health Report 2000.* WHO, Geneva.

26 Xingzhu L (2003) *Policy Tools for Allocative Efficiency of Health Services.* WHO, Geneva.

27 Irwen A and Scali E (2005) *Action on the Social Determinants of Health: learning from previous experiences.* WHO Commission on Social Determinants of Health, Geneva.

Chapter 10

Where is general practice heading?

Summary

In this chapter I describe the story of general practice. This role originated in specialist medical or surgical care and, for this reason, carries a main aim to diagnose and remove diseases. For many years general practice was left to find its own way separately from hospital care. This resulted in the idea that general practitioners (GPs) help patients and their families with all aspects of their health. It is associated with the term 'primary care', which became prominent in the UK after the 1990 health care reforms when multi-disciplinary teams became common in general practice. It is the main medical discipline to have regular and ongoing contact with a complete breadth of other disciplines in health care in the community, and, for this reason, could provide a valuable contribution to shared leadership for integrated health and social care, both horizontally and vertically. Overwhelming demands and strong allegiance to linear ideas about science, health and change make this unrealistic without new skills of systems thinking and practice, new kinds of whole-system support and leadership, and new approaches to multi-disciplinary team-working.

Origins of general practice: 1858–1948

The term 'general practitioner' came into widespread use around the beginning of the nineteenth century and it marked the end of two centuries during which the organisation of medical care had hardly altered. Until then, 'gentlemen' physicians (the Royal College of Physicians was founded in 1518), craftsmen surgeons (the Society of Barber-surgeons was founded in 1540) and tradesmen apothecaries (the Society of Apothecaries was founded in 1617) were clearly distinct kinds of doctor, separated primarily by social class. The GP role arose from each of these traditions but, primarily, general practice work was surgical (hence the GP's surgery) and membership of the Royal College of Surgeons was considered to be the standard qualification.[1]

The Medical Registration Act of 1858 aimed to 'end the evils of a rampant quackery and illegal practice, the absence of uniformity in training or examination and the jealousies, antipathies and hostilities between the members of the profession'.[2] This led to the Medical Register, which distinguished the qualified from the unqualified. There was no real distinction between the consultant and the GP at that time, except that GPs called in consultants. This led to the hospital becoming the domain of the consultant while the GP developed a gate-keeping role to them. This separated the consultant and the GP at the hospital door and removed the GP from the teaching of medical students.[1] It also meant that the advances in medical care which occurred at the end of the nineteenth century and for most of the twentieth century happened almost exclusively in hospitals. It was through this that the different roles of specialist and generalist evolved, and with it the perception in hospital circles that the GP was a second-class doctor. However, the perception in the population was different and the GP was considered to be an important part of the community. It seems that the 'Dr Finlay' image has been evident from early days where the 'family doctor' is interested in, and contributes to, the everyday unfolding of people's life stories, as the following quote from the writings of John Hunt demonstrates:[3]

> As Collings pointed out, we cannot expect to recapture the twentieth century concept of the nineteenth century family physician – benign, bewhiskered, and beloved, with his silk hat and frock coat, leisurely driving round his practice, treating most of his sick patients himself and referring few to hospital . . . Why were so many of them so highly regarded at the time? It was largely because of their strength of character, kindliness, clinical acumen, and wisdom in applying their often empirical knowledge. The deep insight into family life and character remains paramount to this day, so that his role as friend and adviser may still far outweigh, in importance to some families, his purely medical responsibilities. (p. 258)

The scientific rigour that is presently associated with the medical profession owes much to Osler, who, in 1913, emphasised clinical inquisitiveness, the pursuit of personal excellence and the use of scientific method. This has ever since been valued as a central feature of medical professionalism and this tradition continued with general practice as it became more organised from the mid 1960s.[1]

The problems of diseases naturally preoccupied early twentieth-century health workers. It seems strange now to remember that, between 1918 and 1919, 20 million people died worldwide from influenza, more than all those killed in the First World War. Slight infections could be deadly. The physical health of the population generally was not good and the health visitor role came into being as a response to the poor health of soldiers conscripted for the Boer War. Antibiotics were not discovered until 1935 and a widespread acceptance of the connection between disease, nutrition and bodily defences was not made until much later. General practice naturally adapted to this reality and focused on the treatment of diseases in individuals.

From diseases, to whole people in families and communities: 1948–1978

When the National Health Service (NHS) was formed in 1948 in a spirit of post-war enthusiasm, health was understandably considered to be synonymous with freedom from the diseases that caused so much distress. It was felt that technology would, in time, find a cure for everything. Negotiations at that time only partly incorporated GPs in the health service and they remained 'independent contractors', paid by the number of patients on their 'list' (the 'panel' was the forerunner of the 'list' and was started in 1911 as a facility to look after low-wage workers).

The independent contractor status kept general practice isolated from developments in the hospital sector, denying it funds for the technological developments which led to notable advancement of hospital medicine. It was left to visionary leaders from within general practice to establish the profession and this entrepreneurial spirit remains to this day. Before the Family Doctor Charter in 1966 there were barely any new resources for general practice. The Charter acknowledged that infrastructure was needed to help GPs do their job well. Rental of premises was reimbursed, 70% of some staff costs were paid by the Family Practitioner Committee, seniority payments and payments to trainers began. The vocational training scheme for young practitioners started in 1968, post-graduate centres began to end the education isolation of GPs and health authorities started to attach staff to some general practices. The College of General Practitioners, established in 1952, received its Royal charter in 1967. General practice began to be treated seriously.

There were a number of reasons for this, not the least of which was the recognition that common diseases need to be treated effectively, as shown in this 1972 quote from Fry:[2]

> Primary medical care, or general practice in the British context, as the stage of first professional contact in care, represents the diseases and problems that the public consider require skilled health and advice .
> It is surprising how similar is the work of primary care throughout the world. The common diseases are similar, that is, respiratory infections, emotional problems, gastrointestinal disorders, skin diseases and degenerative disorders. (p. 36)

But in the 1970s there was growing criticism of the whole medical industry. The preoccupation of the medical profession with the cure of diseases, scientific method and a 'doctor knows best' attitude was perceived to be de-humanising and promoting of ill-health.[4] One aspect of health – disease – was filtered out by medicine, paying scant attention to other aspects. This became labelled the 'therapeutic era'[5] to denote the dominance of the pharmaceutical industry.

By the late 1970s there was emerging a consensus in general practice that health is more than disease and it is the generalist's role to promote a holistic view of health, as the following quotes from *Trends in General Practice*, 1977, show:[2]

> About Child Care, by Margaret Pollack: 'Services provided for children by general practitioners now include not only traditional medical care, but also psycho-social care of a child within a family group . . . involvement in a team approach with nurses and health visitors attached to the practices . . . by practising preventative medicine can made a contribution to the health and happiness of children in his practice. He is offering a personal service to his patients who, in return, identify him as a person.'

> About the Elderly, by Keith Thomson: 'The role the general practitioner as the co-ordinator of health care for the elderly is certain to become a dominant part of future general practice.'

> About Fertility and Family Medicine, by John McEwan: 'Whatever extent a practitioner may develop and practice his expertise in contra-

ceptive care, there is a second role for the family doctor, with a more fundamental and universal quality: his involvement as an informed advisor in questions of family fertility. The associations between poverty, ill health and large families . . . [it is] firmly part of the family doctor's job to be concerned with family size, family spacing and the prevention of unwanted pregnancies.'

This marked a new distinction between the generalist and the specialist – no longer the geographical separation of a hospital door but a concern for all aspects of health of individuals and families. The GP is still expected to be competent at disease management but this traditional view became complemented with the image of a generalist health worker who is concerned with all aspects of health of the list of people they serve. These quotes suggest a growing awareness that it was natural for the GP to take a role in realising the Alma Ata vision of 'health for all', which was announced the following year and given considerable coverage in the *British Journal of General Practice*.

From practitioners to practices, institutions, networks and systems: 1978–2006

Despite early efforts at community oriented primary care[6] the holistic role claimed by the GP was not matched by the organisational capacity to enact it. A complex co-ordination of multi-disciplinary team-working and systems thinking is needed. It is only in recent years that the UK health care system is developing this potential.

Building from *Promoting Better Health* (1987), *Working for Patients* (1989) and *Caring for People* (1989) a flurry of governmental White Papers in the 1990s provided rhetoric to advance what increasingly became called 'primary care' (ironically, policy makers claimed that the word *health* was too narrow and equated with disease). The 1990 GP new contract introduced screening for disease in general practice. *The Health of the Nation – a Strategy for Public Health in England*, promoted positive health and illness prevention (1992). *The Patients' Charter* emphasised the rights of individual citizens to health care (1992). The *Primary Care Led NHS* (1995), *Primary Care: the Future* (1996), *The NHS: a Service with Ambitions* (1996) and the *Primary Care Act* (1997) all voiced the intention to put a collaborative multi-disciplinary and comprehensive primary care at the centre of the NHS.

The 1990s in the UK brought into view the general practice organisation. Before then everyone talked and thought about GPs. Suddenly, almost overnight and without a fuss, everyone talked about 'general practice'.

There was an obvious reason for this – the team got bigger. To meet requirements for health promotion and the holding of budgets for funding secondary care services there was a need to employ new staff. With the attachment of allied professionals, the extended practice team became the norm. Health Education Authority teambuilding workshops were enthusiastically embraced. Fund-holding abruptly focused practitioner minds on the power of the organisation. Organisational development came to general practice.

Acceleration for the idea of integrated primary health care came from the discovery that generalist care from a community base was more cost effective and efficient than specialist models. The groundbreaking work of Barbara Starfield brought this into sharp focus.[7] She developed a score to measure a country for the strength of their orientation to primary health care as envisaged in the 1996 Ljubljana Charter. She compared the scores of many countries to show a strong association between 'low-cost–high-health' and policy that scored high for primary health care orientation. The escalation of costs in the hospital sector plus recognition that primary health care might be economic and effective, led to a resurgence in the idea of comprehensive primary health care at the same time that the WHO, under the influence of the World Bank, seemed to give up on the idea.

A change to a Labour government in 1997 continued the rhetoric of a 'primary care-led NHS', but also promised attention to the processes of integration. *The New NHS, Modern, Dependable* (1997) stated 'the basis for a 10 year programme to improve the NHS . . . [by] a replacement of the internal market by a system of integrated care'.

The NHS Plan (2000) continued the theme of integration:[8,9]

> *The NHS Plan* sets out an ambitious, 10-year programme of modernisation for health and social services which will provide patients with a uniformly high standard of service fit for the 21st century. *The NHS Plan* sets out the Government's intention to move towards local ownership of targets and freedoms to innovate within a clear framework of accountability.

Primary Care Act pilot schemes, primary care groups, health action zones, new deals for communities, health improvement plans – all advanced ideas about organisational capacity for integrated primary care.

The growth in organisational capacity brought with it a conflict of values.[10] Practices were expected to operate as a coherent unit to improve the health of the whole population, as well as care for the individuals who presented with problems. These different priorities demand different actions. The new GP contract of 2004 brought this conflict into further relief – it was located with the general practice organisation rather than with individual practitioners.

The story of general practice was taking new direction. It had evolved out of hospital medical care into whole-person family care. It was now about to explore the territory of whole-population care – public health.

Three different kinds of organisation

An organisation is 'a group of people formed into a society, union or a business' (*Chambers 21st Century Dictionary*). It can be any grouping of people that has an agreed way to organise their relationships. Different kinds of organisation shape these relationships differently.

General practices are small enterprises

The organisation of general practice is a small enterprise, employing no more than 50 people. This makes it possible to retain a sense of family, where everyone knows everyone else and what they do. Authority is exercised by a group of 'partners' who interpret the rules, often in an ad hoc and informal way. The shared mission is the care of the (1000–20 000) patients on the practice 'list'.

Patients can choose to belong to any practice within a certain area that has an open list. UK NHS treatment is funded through general taxation, so practitioners treat patients according to need rather than the idiosyncrasies of different insurance policies. General practice acts as a gateway to other medical services. Most of these are also funded through taxation.

Primary care organisations are co-ordinating or networking institutions

In contrast, PCOs are large institutions with a co-ordinating role, employing large numbers of people and relating to a local health economy which includes other institutions such as hospitals. Their size mandates bureaucratic structures of line management and written organisational rules. They offer the structural opportunity to bring together general practices and other local organisations and disciplines. This could result in multi-disciplinary participation for co-ordinated primary health care that has not previously been a realistic option. However, only 3% of the budget is allocated to management and this may be insufficient to realise this ambitious role.

Networks connect a variety of organisations and individuals

At the same time there has developed a strong emphasis on the use of networks to stimulate innovation throughout large areas. A network is a form of organisation that connects people from a variety of organisations. It has no authority except the power of persuasion and the contracts made between network members. Enquiry through networks can facilitate innovation between bureaucracies that more usually stifle innovation.[11] Networked activity will be needed to develop 'enhanced services' for conditions such as mental illness, and 'practice-based commissioning' (commissioning for services will be devolved to PCO localities). 'Intermediate care' will need network thinking to develop care pathways shared between primary and secondary care. Clinical and research networks will broker academic/practitioner partnerships.

Thus, for generations GPs have worked outside organisations. Within 15 years this has changed and they now relate intimately to three different organisational forms: a small enterprise (the practice); large institutions (PCOs); and a variety of networks.

A similar steep learning curve faces other semi-independent practitioners in primary care, such as dentists and pharmacists.

Choices for future general practice?

Placing general practice centre-stage requires us to describe what it is we do. Before, we could muddle through doing what felt right, but calling it a mystery.[12]

One consequence of this has been a growing interest in complexity theory[13,14] and narrative.[15,16] These provide practitioners with explanatory models for the complex adaptivity of human beings evolving together within multiple interconnected communities. The roles are multiple. As Hellman puts it:[17]

> the modern GP has multiple, often contradictory roles – not only as medical scientist, but also as educator, priest, beautician, government representative, researcher, marriage guidance counsellor, psychotherapist, pharmacist, friend, relative, financial adviser, as well as

anthropologist – intimately familiar with the local community, its needs, traditions, dialects, and ethnic composition.

Outside the GP's door, facilitators and advisers wait to advise on each aspect. And paralysis by paper has developed as the scientific evidence for everything that lands in the lap of GPs. To deal with new contract requirements energies have become focused on chronic disease management, computer systems and emotional survival. The issues inherent to the more intangible aspects of being a generalist are temporarily put aside.

But where lies the future of general medical practice?

On the face of it there is a choice – general practice can specialise in vertical integration with hospital specialists (as required for a disease approach to health care) or in horizontal integration with other community practitioners (as required for a community approach).

But to be true to our heritage there is no meaningful choice here. Both are needed. Losing medical integration would prevent treating diseases properly. Losing multi-disciplinary community integration would prevent treating people properly.

This is more than any individual can ever do alone. If general practice is to survive there needs to develop sophisticated systems of support to achieve and maintain the breadth of required competencies. Both horizontal and vertical integration can be supported by computers and by facilitative approaches to human interaction. Computers can help visualise care pathways vertically and service options laterally. Facilitation can help primary secondary care to interface vertically and multi-disciplinary team-working horizontally.

These competencies include the following.

- GPs need to be medically competent – they need to be competent in the identification of diseases from A to Z in medical textbooks, and know what to do about them. This requires a level of computer decision support greater than anything so far achieved, as well as skills to systematically learn from experience.[18,19]

- GPs need to be competent in the consulting room – they need to be able to surface and deal with a breadth of problems, and help patients to make sense of these in the light of their overall life stories. This requires the development of consulting skills which help patients to recognise and improve their narratives,[16] not so much 'doctor-centred' or 'patient-centred', but centred on the coherence of someone's life story, helped by trusted relationships and reflective practice.

- GPs need to be systems and team competent – they need to understand how to be effective members of different kinds of organisation and different teams, and what things will help whole systems to learn and change. This requires becoming systems practitioners, skilled at dealing with soft, hard and whole systems. It requires team-working in small organisations, large institutions and networks.

- GPs need to be epistemologically aware – they need to be competent at evaluating and generating different kinds of knowledge, and using these wisely in different contexts. The limitation of words and theories needs to be recognised. A science of listening and reflection needs to be better described.

Continuing professional development support can help practitioners with these competencies.

Implications for primary care organisations

GPs face a steep learning curve. Integrated primary health care challenges a long tradition of working on a one-to-one basis, outside organisations. A co-ordinated set of learning opportunities is needed to work well within these new organisational structures. Chapter 13 describes ways to think about organisational learning. Chapter 5 describes practical things to do when facilitating learning spaces.

GPs are potentially valuable contributors to whole-system integration, because the role reaches into all parts of health and social care. Opportunities to experience shared leadership through networks and localities are needed. Chapter 13 describes practical policy for PCOs to develop this. Chapter 6 suggests how to strategically place networks.

The strong adherence of medical practice to positivist approaches to enquiry and linear approaches to change may prevent progress. Epistemological awareness needs to be taught and modelled by those who lead learning, audit and research (Chapter 11). Chapter 7 describes how to bring together an appropriate breadth of knowledge.

References

1 Tudor Hart J (1988) *A New Kind of Doctor*. Merlin Press, London.
2 Louden I, Fry J, Howie J, Pollak M, Thompson K, Lloyd G *et al.* (1977) *Trends in General Practice*. Royal College of General Practitioners, London.
3 Hunt J (1992) *The Writings of John Hunt*. Royal College of General Practitioners, Exeter.
4 Illich I (1970) *Medical Nemesis – the Expropriation of Health* . . . Pantheon Books, New York (1976 edition).
5 Ashton J and Seymour H (1988) *The New Public Health*. Open University Press, Buckingham.
6 Nutting PA (1987) *Community Oriented Primary Care: from principle to practice*. US Department of Health and Human Sciences, Office of Primary Care Studies, Washington, DC.
7 Starfield B (1998) *Primary Care – Balancing Health Needs, Services and Technology*. Oxford University Press, Oxford.
8 NHS Executive (2001) *The NHS Plan – Implementing the Performance Improvement Agenda – A Policy Position Statement and Consultation Document*. NHS Executive, London.
9 Secretary of State for Health (2000) *The NHS Plan: a plan for investment; a plan for reform*. Cm 4818-I. 2000. HMSO, London.
10 Pratt J (1995) *Practitioners and Practices – A Conflict of Values?* Radcliffe Medical Press, Oxford.
11 Thomas P, McDonnell J, McCulloch J, While A, Bosanquet N and Ferlie E (2005) Increasing capacity for innovation in large bureaucratic primary care organizations – a whole system participatory action research project. *Annals of Family Medicine*. 3: 312–17.
12 Heath I (1995) *The Mystery of General Practice*. Nuffield Provincial Hospitals Trust, London.
13 Griffiths F and Byrne D (1999) General practice and the new science emerging from the theories of 'chaos' and complexity. *British Journal of General Practice*. 48: 1697–9.

14 Kernick D (2004) *Complexity and Health Care Organisation – A View from the Street.* Radcliffe Medical Press, Oxford.
15 Greenhalgh T and Hurwitz B (1998) *Narrative Based Medicine.* BMJ Publications, London.
16 Launer J (2002) *Narrative-based Primary Care. A Practical Guide.* Radcliffe Medical Press, Oxford.
17 Helman C (2002) The culture of general practice. *British Journal of General Practice.* **52**: 619–20.
18 Stanley I, Al Shehr A and Thomas P (1993) Continuing education for general practitioners 2: systematic learning from experience. *British Journal of General Practice.* **43**: 249–53.
19 Stanley I, Al Shehr A and Thomas P (1993) Continuing education for general practitioners 1: experience, competence, and the media of self directed learning for established general practitioners. *British Journal of General Practice.* **43**: 210–14.

Chapter 11

Towards an integrating theory of knowledge

My thanks to John Horder, Peter Kinch, Will Miller, Mike Parker and Kurt Stange, for their help with presenting the ideas in this chapter. A modified version appears in the *Annals of Family Medicine* Vol 4 No. 5 2006. www.Amfammed.org

Summary

In this chapter I challenge the central relevance of traditional (positivist) objective science to the complexities experienced on a daily basis by generalist practice, and to effective learning and change. I suggest that 'critical theory' and 'constructivism' offer equally valid and useful lenses with which to view the world. They relate to qualitative and participatory approaches to enquiry. Second, I argue that knowledge generated by any of these approaches is not truth itself, but a snapshot of more complex and moving stories. To reveal a trustworthy picture knowledge must make sense of whole stories. A combination of all three approaches to the generation of knowledge is needed, often at the same time.

Primary care practitioners and researchers are largely expected to explain our work with patients in ways which stem from 'positivism' – a school of philosophy that maintains that knowledge can only come from observable phenomena and positive facts (*Chambers 21st Century Dictionary*). It does this wherever possible in quantitative terms. This reveals a thin and static world, and it holds us back from describing more complex phenomena and gaining genuinely new insights. Evidence generated in this way can never fully represent a situation. It is better understood as a snapshot taken at one moment in the course of a complex, evolving story.

But the same practitioners and researchers habitually draw on two other theories of knowledge besides positivism, to make sense of patients' health and illnesses. These are 'critical theory' and 'constructivism'. Both lead to qualitative and participatory approaches to enquiry. Better understanding of the strengths and weaknesses of all three theories will allow us to do our clinical work better and to frame an approach to research that can better reveal its multi-faceted and changing aspects. Below, I use a clinical case to show that we already use these three theories in everyday practice. Later, I analyse their distinctive features. Lastly, I argue that each approach has strengths and weaknesses. The ideal is a combination of all three.

A brief clinical encounter

The case is of a man I saw at home. He was the patient of another doctor and I did not see him again. This makes it easier for me to focus on what kind of knowledge I was working with in-the-moment, rather than telling the story with hindsight, after a diagnosis had been reached.

He was an elderly black African man. His diabetes was well controlled. He complained of a painful toe that his usual physician had reviewed several times. In view of his good foot pulses and identical appearance of his toes, I was initially inclined to agree with his usual doctor that this was not a sign of ischaemia (poor blood flow to the toe). I observed the pictures on the wall of him as a younger man dancing and compared this with the barely mobile person in front of me. I asked him to tell me his story and what sense he made of it. He told me that this toe had 'gone black'; he was worried that his toes would have to be amputated, as had happened to his mother.

I considered alternative explanations. I knew that a blackening toe can be a sign of serious ischaemia. I entertained the idea that he could see a different version of black that I could not – he was, after all, very dark-skinned and my eyes may not be adequately attuned. Also, the toe was clearly painful and there was no adequate explanation for this. I also wondered whether there were other things affecting his health which had not surfaced – perhaps he mourned the loss of his athletic youth, or had unresolved issues to do with his mother. This prompted me to chat more generally, searching for concerns unrelated to the toe. He disclosed his intense loneliness. He started to say more, then drew back, indicating with his hand for me to change the subject. I paused before I asked him what we should do. He wanted tests on his toe. I agreed to ask his usual doctor to arrange this. He could speak about the other things on another day.

What different kinds of enquiry was I using in this encounter? And what knowledge did they generate? First, I undertook a clinical examination. This aimed to identify observable evidence of a disease process in his painful toe – I found none. Second, I listened to him. Through this, through observations and through open questions that allowed him to speak in his own terms, I aimed to get beyond my pre-judgements and reliance on objective evidence to explore interpretations I had not initially considered. I asked him his views, considered the relevance of photographs, and observed the way he carried himself and talked about other issues. This resulted in the new insight of his loneliness and paved the way for a different kind of conversation next time. Third, I reflected on the experience of this encounter in the light of other clinical encounters from my past, to detect patterns that I recognised. I also reflected the patterns I recognised against patterns he recognised (his mother's amputated toes) to establish a shared explanatory model with which to make decisions about next steps (referral for tests).

When I did the clinical examination I was drawing on the 'positivist' tradition to find objective evidence of ischaemia. When I listened to him I was drawing on a 'critical theory' tradition of qualitative research. When I reflected this experience against other experiences I was drawing on the 'constructivist' tradition that reveals connections between different things. I did not pause to consider what enquiry I was using at any one time, nor did I use them sequentially. Instead, I rapidly shifted between all three approaches to clarify his narrative,[1] and find a coherent or believable fit between the different kinds of knowledge being generated – before I went to the next home visit.

My training leads me to believe that the central task of a physician is the objective assessment of a problem to move towards a diagnosis. In this encounter the linear 'problem–objective assessment–diagnosis' model did not help me to make a decision about what to do next. It also did not help me to see other aspects of his health that I might be able to help. I used listening and reflection not to reinforce my own prejudgements, but as enquiries in their own right. These generated insights and a shared explanatory model with which to move forward.

In the next section I analyse the nature and limitations of knowledge generated through these three paradigms in order to argue that they are complementary – all are needed.

Positivism, critical theory and constructivism reveal different kinds of insight

> A man dropped his watch in a dark street and asked passers by to search for it with him under the street lamp. 'Where did you drop it?' asked one. 'Over there,' said the man. 'Then why are you looking here?' The man replied, 'Because this is where the light is.'

In this section I suggest that positivism, critical theory and constructivism reflect three fundamentally different and complementary ways of illuminating the world. They can throw light in different places and reveal different things.

The things that are revealed are different because each gives a different combination of answers to the following three questions:

• What is the nature of 'reality', or the 'knowable'? (an ontological question).
• What is the nature of the relationship between the enquirer and the knowable? (an epistemological question).
• How should the enquirer go about finding out knowledge (a methodological question).[2]

Positivism is the dominant paradigm in medicine. It expects the world to be simply ordered and predictable. Change happens through a simple linear process of cause and effect. It believes a 'realist ontology'[2] – something 'really exists' unchanging and irrespective of other things. Something is objectively and undeniably there in isolation, like a nugget of gold waiting to be mined. Its epistemology is dualist/objectivist – 'it is either there or not'. Its methodology is experimental/manipulative – 'a question/hypothesis is stated in advance in propositional form and subjected to empirical tests under controlled conditions'.[2] We use positivism in quantitative research such as randomised controlled trials, where features of interest are named in advance and counted. Validity requires statistical difference between numbers. It has no power to reveal connections or context (discrete features are counted in isolation from other things) and no power to reveal novelty (things must be named in advance). I used this approach to examine my patient's toe.

Positivism is the best approach to predict what will happen in simple situations. It gives us reason to trust the structural integrity of aircraft, and agree what forms of treatment are better at curing named diseases. However, it only remains reliable in tightly controlled and slowly changing situations. Complexity theory shows that when different factors interact they adapt to each other, creating new forms and unpredictable directions.[3] Positivism cannot deal with this adaptation and unpredictability. It can analyse what is happening inside a controlled laboratory, but the moving context that swirls around that laboratory is invisible to its eyes.

The recognition that positivism cannot consider hidden factors gave rise to a school of thought called 'critical (social) theory' or 'ideologically oriented inquiry'.[2] It is associated with the German philosopher Jurgen Habermas, who maintained that our understandings of the world are distorted because we are blind to many things of relevance.[4] Contemporary interpretations of critical theory are 'concerned in particular with issues of power and justice and the ways that the economy, matters of race, class and gender, ideologies, discourses, education, religion and other social institutions, and cultural dynamics interact to construct a social system'.[5] Its ontology is 'critical realist' in that truth is still expected to be 'really there', but hidden by more superficial truths.[2] The researcher is challenged to consider different perspectives and meanings that are not immediately obvious. Change happens by overthrowing wrong ideologies. Its epistemology is subjectivist in that it values different interpretations.[2] Its methodology is 'dialogic' – we debate the rights and wrongs of different versions of the truth to remove 'false consciousness', and from this arrive at a better version of the truth.[2] This approach uses research methods such as case studies, which can reveal a rich picture. Validity requires that the picture is 'trustworthy' or useful in other contexts. I used this approach to explore hidden aspects of my patient's health.

This may help to dig deeper but neither positivism nor critical theory has the power to understand 'novelty'. Both assume 'realist ontology' – truth is in there somewhere, already defined and waiting to be found. But this does not describe newly created form. It may be possible to track contributions to something new, but true novelty is created, not found. Flour, raisins, milk and salt may contribute to the baking of a cake; two parents give life to a child. The cake and the child were co-created from various factors, but are not the same thing as those original factors. It is incorrect to imagine that they were already defined and waiting to be discovered. Complexity theorists describe the mechanism of such co-creation as 'complex responsive processes',[6] whereby multiple interactions, competitions and adaptations give rise to new ways forward that could not be predicted at the outset.

True novelty can be explained by 'social constructionism'. This maintains that 'all socially significant dimensions of interaction . . . originate and are constructed in joint action'[7] (p. 179). The related theory of knowledge is termed 'constructivism',[2] and relates to Maturana's idea of autopoiesis – literally 'self-creating'[8] (p. 141). It does not have a 'realist', but a 'relativist ontology'[2] – things are true in as much as the observer is somehow bound up in the co-creation of the truth. It requires us to acknowledge that we 'cannot claim that a reality out there exists independently of ourselves as observers'[8] (p. 141). Change happens through innovative adaptations between different things. Ontology in this theory of knowledge is relativist and epistemology is subjectivist, but the ontological/epistemological distinction is obliterated because what is 'really there', and the relation of the observer to it, are different versions of the same question.[2] Methodology is hermeneutic/dialectic – a dynamic iterative exploration of different meanings (I relate this in Chapter 13 to Bateson's idea of 'deutero-learning' – learning how to learn). This helps diverse insights to become relevant to each other in a process that weaves together different insights to appreciate new ways of thinking and acting. Methods that facilitate this include appreciative enquiry,[9] participatory action research[10] and large group interventions.[11] Validity requires that things make sense as a whole to the people involved. I used this approach to make connections with the connections made by my patient.

My claim is that these three theories of knowledge filter out three equally important aspects of whole situations. Together they help clinicians to rigorously practice a science that sees more of the whole person than their diagnoses. It helps managers to devise complex strategies for change that involve nurturing new ideas, and participation of stakeholders in co-creative processes, to complement 'top down' directives. It helps leaders of research and audit to decide what combination of research approaches will best answer the questions that interest them, and best result in their findings being appropriately used.

In the next section I will argue that most situations encountered by practitioners, managers and researchers in primary care are helped by the simultaneous use of all three paradigms, and the result is 'common sense'.

What you see depends on how you look

> One scientist to another: 'I've had a terrible day. Someone broke into the lab last night and the mice just aren't doing what they are supposed to do.'

A theory is 'a series of ideas which seek to explain some aspect of the world' (*Chambers 21st Century Dictionary*). It is not intended to reveal everything – merely 'some aspect'. Positivism, critical theory and constructivism are basic theories. They, too, highlight an aspect – an aspect of a whole situation that resonates with their assumptions about what there is to see (ontology) and how they look (methodology). Other aspects influencing behaviour within the whole situation will be invisible to these eyes.

The interdependence of what you see and how you look is evidenced in daily experience. As a gardener, when I 'look' at a garden with my ears I hear bird song. If I look with my nose I smell flower pollen. Each sense filters out from a whole picture the aspect that connects with the way I am looking. If I look with the eyes of positivism I will see things that can be named and counted – trees and birds. If I look with the eyes of critical theory I will see hidden things – soil substructure and territory guarded by a robin. If I look with the eyes of constructivism I will see dynamic interactions between different things – the response of birds to a cat or the changing seasons. No basic theory can allow one to see it all.

Each paradigm of inquiry has advantages and disadvantages, summarised in Table 11.1 below.

Table 11.1 Paradigms of enquiry

	Advantages	Disadvantages
Positivism	Can predict what will happen in simple situations	Tends to overly simplistic interpretations and short-term goals
Critical theory	Reveals hidden factors and different perspectives in complex situations	Tends to time-consuming analysis of irreconcilable viewpoints
Constructivism	Facilitates innovation and shared understanding	Tends to slow processes of consensus-creation, without focus

The advantage of using all three together is to see a rich picture with which better decisions can be made. To appreciate the garden as a whole the gardener will use all senses to 'see' a rich picture. To appreciate a whole person or whole situation practitioners, managers and researchers can likewise use all three ways of enquiring. In some situations one narrow insight is adequate. With my patient, a test was the way to resolve doubts about ischaemia. In other consultations priorities are less clear. For example, patients with multiple problems, physical disabilities and mental health problems commonly experience mismatch between objective evidence and subjective feelings. The experienced practitioner knows that these situations require careful exploration of various factors, and negotiation of the best plan.

The value of using complementary research approaches in primary care is no longer contentious.[12] The validity of their conclusions is.[13] There is an epistemological problem here – many people assume that scientific evidence or knowledge is truth itself, rather than an insight into more connected and evolving truths. This leads to arguments about who is right and who is wrong, when a better course of action would be to explore the value of different perspectives, and crystallise[14,15] from them what they mean for action in their specific context.

An epistemology of common sense

To be epistemologically naive is to believe that knowledge can be isolated from context. To be epistemologically aware is to recognise that knowledge is bound by the context of its generation, and what you see depends on how you look. Knowledge illuminates aspects of complex and co-evolving stories, but its relevance in other contexts cannot be assumed.[16,17]

The idea I am putting forward is that evidence and theories are not 'truth' itself but lenses that filter certain things out from complexity. They say at least as much about what we are able to see as about what there is to be seen. Similarly positivism, critical theory and constructivism say at least as much about how our minds construct ideas as they do about laws of nature. It is not a new idea. Heisenberg said: 'what we observe is not nature itself, but nature exposed to our method of questioning'.[18]

The idea I am putting forward suggests that what we know about the past contributes to, but does not predict, the future. This, too, is not a new idea. Kierkegaard said:

Most organizational theorists, as well as most philosophers, mistake the certainty of structures seen in hindsight for the emergent order that frames living forward. Neither group of scholars has come to grips with the fact that their conceptual understandings trail life and are of a different character than is living forward.[19]

I am putting forward an 'epistemology of common sense'. 'Common sense' comes from the same linguistic root as *consensus*, from the Latin *consentire* – to agree. Insights from different enquiries must 'make sense in common' with those who are experiencing the lived-reality. For individuals to comfortably embrace a proposed way forward it must also fit with their personal beliefs and with the culture of the groups to which they belong (Chapter 1). Common sense is not one simple thing, but a dance between different beliefs, priorities and needs, to find a workable fit that those involved can go along with. It uses all three theories of knowledge – constructivism, positivism and critical theory – to feel that a proposal is grounded in both objective and subjective reality. Common sense recognises that different combinations will be needed on different days for different reasons.

Implications for primary care practice, management and enquiry

This analysis puts primary care practitioners, managers and researchers into a place of uncertainty. In each situation they will have a sense of what they know, but be largely unaware of what they don't know. Skills of living with uncertainty may be needed.

Practitioners will be more familiar with positivist approaches to enquiry. Complementary qualitative and participatory audit and research need to be also learnt and valued, and rigorous ways developed to bring together different research insights.

Being skilled at weaving together positivism, critical theory and constructivism will reveal a rich picture for practitioners and managers. PCOs need to support the development of whole sectors as case studies of health service delivery, providing opportunities for different research and audit teams to interact. They need to develop to bring together multiple insights about whole sectors.

Some say that simultaneously using three different approaches to enquiry is too difficult to act on. I disagree. In 1993 in Liverpool a coalition of authorities agreed that practices, as multi-disciplinary teams, must write and perform audits of 'quantity, quality and consensus' to achieve the highest level of payments for health promotion. Supported by facilitators 80% of the 110 practices in the city did this – and they enjoyed it.

The stakes are high. Unopposed linear thinking, given credence by positivism, threatens the very existence of generalist practice – medical and non-medical. It promotes unthinking application of evidence, simplistic approaches to change, and research that avoids the most difficult issues. In the consulting room, in management, and in all manner of enquiry it needs to be complemented by disciplined and rigorous consideration of complementary ways of thinking and acting.

References

1 Launer J (2002) *Narrative-based Primary Care. A Practical Guide*. Radcliffe Medical Press, Oxford.
2 Guba E (1990) *The Paradigm Dialog*. Sage, Newbury Park, CA.
3 Kernick D (2004) *Complexity and Health Care Organisation – A View from the Street*. Radcliffe Medical Press, Abingdon.
4 Wulff H, Pederson A and Rosenburg R (1990) *Philosophy of Medicine – An Introduction*. Blackwell, Oxford.
5 Kincheloe JL and McLaren P (2000) Rethinking critical theory and qualitative research. In: N Denzin and Y Lincoln (eds) *Handbook of Qualitative Research*. Sage, Thousand Oaks, CA.
6 Stacey R (2001) *Complex Responsive Processes in Organizations*. Routledge, London.
7 Shotter J (2000) *Conversational Realities – Constructing Life through Language*. Sage, London.
8 Carr A (2000) Theories that focus on belief systems. In: A Carr (ed) *Family Therapy. Concepts, Processes and Practice*. John Wiley, London.
9 Whitney D and Trosten-Bloom A (2003) *The Power of Appreciative Inquiry*. Berrett-Koehler, San Francisco, CA.
10 Whyte WF (1991) *Participatory Action Research*. Sage, New York, NY.
11 Benedict BB and Alban B (1997) *Large Group Interventions – Engaging the Whole System for Rapid Change*. Jossey-Bass, San Francisco, CA.
12 Stange K (2004) In this issue: multimethod research. *Annals of Family Medicine*. **2**: 2–3.
13 Borkan JM (2004) Mixed methods studies: a foundation for primary care research. *Annals of Family Medicine*. **2**: 4–6.
14 Janesick VJ (2000) The choreography of qualitative research design. In: N Denzin and Y Lincoln (eds) *Handbook of Qualitative Research*. Sage, Thousand Oaks, CA.
15 Kemmis S and McTaggart R (2000) Participatory action research. In: N Denzin and Y Lincoln (eds) *Handbook of Qualitative Research*. Sage, Thousand Oaks, CA.
16 Kravtitz RL, Duan N and Braslow J (2004) Evidence-based medicine, heterogeneity of treatment effects, and the trouble with averages. *The Milbank Quarterly*. **82**: 661–87.
17 Rothwell PM (2005) External validity of randomised controlled trials: 'To whom do the results of this trial apply?' *Lancet*. **365**: 82–93.
18 Capra F (1997) *The Web of Life*. Flamingo, London.
19 Weick KE (1999) That's moving: theories that matter. *Journal of Management Inquiry*. **8**: 134–42.

Chapter 12

Towards an integrating theory of health

Summary

In this chapter, I consider the meaning of health in the light of the limitations of theories described in Chapter 11. Health is what people need to develop a life story that is meaningful to them. Clearly, diseases affect how a life story will evolve, but they are not the same thing as, and are less important than, the overall story. People seek 'narrative unity' – a coherent life story in which they are the lead actor, and which shapes their sense of self. Motivation for change comes from multiple hidden factors within these stories and the web of relationships that validates them. Change that is more than superficial alters their web of relationships and will be enthusiastically embraced if they can see how it might enhance the coherence of the story.

On my left was Roberto, a stocky, stern-faced Navajo man. On my right walked Elaine, a tall, thin Afro-American woman on vacation far west from her Atlanta home. The ease with which we felt each other's presence might have made an onlooker imagine that we were old friends. But there were no onlookers – the canyon was empty. It was January 1996.

In truth we had known each other for less than an hour, and within two hours we would part without even taking each other's addresses. We didn't even ask permission to walk together. We sort of fell in with each other, feeling mutual assent, having paused at the same high spot to view the breathtaking dusty-brown plunging slopes – a cowboy movie-set without the actors. Silently we picked our way down the thin path to the canyon floor where a nearly dry stream gave life to some scrubby trees.

Roberto spoke: 'Here, Kit Carson led the troops that enslaved the Navajo nation. I come here to remember.' This action, in 1864, led to the 'long walk': 8000 men, women and children were forced to walk 300 miles to New Mexico where they were held in captivity. Roberto explained that he lived nearby with his wife and child; he worked in a factory making artefacts for tourists. Almost every week he walked the canyon.

We walked on.

I told them that I had been developing multi-disciplinary general practice in England. There was no easy next step for me, so I had accepted a post in South Africa to continue my work. I was travelling for a few months to catch my breath before I started a whole new life.

The air was clear. It was warm but not hot. The sense of history was strong. Each of us was deeply conscious of our own story, and how it connected with other, bigger stories. We had nothing in common with each other, and everything in common – both at the same time.

Elaine said 'We are all many things. And each carries its own history. I am Afro-American; and I am African. I am also a health visitor and a citizen of the world. These are all true, at the same time; and each makes different demands of me, and involves me in different stories.'

Health is the foundation for achievement

The word *health* originates from the Old English *haelth* and the Germani *hal*, and relates to the word *whole* (*Chambers 21st Century Dictionary* 1999). Boorse describes health as 'normal species function'.[1] This definition demonstrates that the meaning of health depends on who we think we are. It demands the speaker to define *who* is deciding *what* as 'normal'.

Seedhouse explored the adequacy of different definitions of health and found them all wanting. The Alma Ata definition of health as an ideal state is 'well-meaning rhetoric'; Talcott Parsons' definition that health is physical and mental fitness to perform socialised daily tasks is 'too narrow'. Health as a commodity, the dominant image in UK health care, 'conceals from people their wider potential by undermining their metaphysical strengths'. Each of these definitions of health has its use but none says it all. Seedhouse concludes that health is 'the foundation for achievement'.[2] Health is a cluster of things that help people to achieve their meaningful future.

Roberto, Elaine and I used our health to walk through the Canyon de Chelly. We needed physical health to walk, and social health to engage with each other. We needed mental health to interpret what each other said. We needed spiritual health to feel 'an aliveness of body and mind as a unity'[3] – the connections between the different dimensions of health. Health is what we needed to develop our own meaningful life stories. We each drew on this to make sense of the moment.

The meaning of meaning

In the book, *Life and Meaning – A Reader*, 29 philosophers discuss meaning in short chapters.[4] Early chapters put forward essentialist theory – theory of the 'essential' nature of man [*sic*]. This theory argues that meaning has already been decided by a higher authority and it is inside there somewhere waiting to be discovered and dug out – the individual finds meaning through discovering and following this pre-ordained path. At any moment 'being good' can involve doing whatever one likes as long as it does not conflict with the rules of the defining authority. Later chapters argue 'existentialist' theory (for example, in the chapter 'Freedom and Bad Faith' by Sartre) where meaning is created out of human interaction in the world. At any one time we are confronted with a number of options and meaning is felt by weaving the best story we can with whatever we have. One of the striking things about these essays is that neither the controlling, dependent 'essential' view of the world nor the boundary-less ever-creating 'existential' view of the world fits with what people I know experience. Everyday life offers both. Also, neither on its own is attractive – mindless dependency and endless existential angst are equally unappealing.

Bringing together what is known and unknown in the present

'Social constructionism' offers an alternative understanding that has place for both essentialism and existentialism.[5] It does this by avoiding a focus on the essentialist or existentialist 'state' and instead focusing on the processes that connect them. The past and the future can be considered to be in constant dialogue with each other in the present moment. Thus 'both the past and the future are other ways of living in the present' (thanks to Ray Ison for this quote). Past and future are constructs that describe where I sit in relation to a developing story. Both past and future can be re-interpreted in the present. For example, with new insights I may tell a different version of a previous experience or change my expectations of the coming year.

The distinction between essentialism, with its clear, simple certainty, and existentialism, which is multifaceted, uncertain and exploratory, recurs in different contexts. Essentialism is 'top down' in that it is pre-conceived and the receiver has only the choices of saying 'yes' or 'no'. It relates to the simple linear and compartmentalised understandings of truth used by positivism. Existentialism is 'bottom up' in that it is exploratory and unknown, open to multiple development directions. It relates to 'critical theory' in that it expects multiple hidden meanings that may include both threats and opportunities. It also relates to 'constructivism' in that it expects change to happen through participation in a creative process.

Essentialism and existentialism are not polarities (although they are often described as such), since they are not the opposite of each other. They are different ways of thinking, one filtering out (past) certainty and the other (future) uncertainty. Here, we find the paradox within the term 'R&D'. 'Re-search' – literally to search again – implies looking backwards at what is 'known'. 'Development' – to grow or to evolve – is a future-looking exercise about what may evolve. I do not mean that there is an unquestionable connection between 'known' and 'past' nor between 'uncertain' and 'future'. What people think they know of the past often turns out to be misleading, and uncertain future can feel very familiar.

If I look with the eyes of essentialism I will see clear simple certainty. If I look with the eyes of existentialism I will see a complex array of opportunities and threats. Both certainty and uncertainty are true at the same time.

But neither is the whole truth, and both can change. But like 'the whole person', or 'the whole story', the whole truth in an absolute sense is unknowable. The 'whole truth' as we know it is limited both by what we are able to 'see' and what we are prepared to see. As Maturana and Varela write: 'the world everyone sees is not *the* world, but *a* world, which we bring forth with others'.[3] So what someone can see of the whole depends on who they are. But how do we get to who we are?

Identity construction

Taylor explores the making of identity and a sense of self.[6] He maintains that 'the self is constituted through exchange in language' (p. 509).

Shotter agrees with this view and maintains that:[5]

> . . . most of the time we do not fully understand what another person says. Indeed in practices, shared understandings occur only occasionally, if they occur at all. And when they do, it is by people testing and checking each others' talk, by them questioning and challenging it, reformulating and elaborating it, and so on . . . Primarily, it seems, they are responding to each other's utterances in an attempt to link their practical activities in with those around them; and in these attempts at co-ordinating their activities, people are constructing one or another kind of social relationship. (p. 2)

This does not mean that growth of identity is itself healthy. Taylor elaborates:[6]

> The fact that the self is constituted through exchange in language (and I strongly agree with Habermas on this) doesn't in any way guarantee us against loss of meaning, fragmentation, the loss of substance in our human environment and our affiliations . . . What gets lost from view here is not the demands of expressive fulfilment . . . [but] the search for moral sources outside the subject through languages which resonate within him or her, the grasping of an order which is inseparably indexed to a personal vision. (p. 509)

This means that every person is actively searching his or her external and internal worlds in search of resonance. Words are used to mark things perceived to be important. For example, they may sense 'this is my sort of person', or 'this is not my sort of person', and then, as a second thought find words to explain why they believe this to be the case. This is a process of both establishing and advancing their sense of self. The 'real-me' is constantly being both discovered and created. These external reference points (good and bad) define an external 'web of relationships'. A similar internal web of reference points (good and bad) defines different aspects of their inner life. These internal and external webs define the 'whole' as perceived by the person – the web-holder.

The 'mysterious' aspects of general practice are concerned with this 'part–whole coherence'. To feel an integrated self, people need to feel that they are a unique person with internal and external cohesion. This does not mean they feel good about themselves or fulfil their potential. It merely means that they feel integrated.

A patient may consult a GP about a discrete problem. They want this to be treated seriously, but they also want the encounter to in some ways enhance their whole sense of self. A GP does this by not merely solving the discrete problem, but by doing it in a way that makes the patient feel a more coherent, empowered and self-aware human being. This may require nothing more than listening carefully then saying something like: 'I think you have done exactly what I would have done and I agree with your analysis (that is if I genuinely do) . . . now here is another thing to think of.'

Communities have a similar need to create part–whole coherence. Shotter again:[5]

> 'the social processes involved', he [Vico] claims, 'are based not upon anything pre-established either in people or their surroundings, but in socially shared identities of feeling they themselves create in the flow of activity between them.' (p. 54)

This leads to a dynamic tension between individual and collective identities. The web of relationships that forms the identity of an individual includes people who share aspects of their identity with others in the same and other webs. They overlap but are not the same thing as the identity of each individual.

People whose worlds of understanding overlap to a considerable extent have a shared identity. This explains the contemporary understanding of 'culture':

> Within the Birmingham School, where the concept of 'cultural studies' originates, the concept of culture has been taken to refer to something like collective subjectivity – that is, a way of life or outlook adopted by a community or social class. This opposes the formerly predominant hierarchic notion, which takes culture as referring to the best and most glorious achievements of a people or civilisation.[7]

Culture is thus a manifestation of shared identity within a community. Multiple sub-communities coexist (in both 'healthy' and 'unhealthy' communities), creating a dense web of interconnections each of which has its own internal coherence.

But why is coherence so important?

Each person is the lead actor in the feature film that is his or her life story

MacIntyre's notion of narrative unity explains the need for coherence. He writes:[8]

> A central thesis then begins to emerge: man in his actions and practice, as well as in his fictions, is essentially a story-telling animal . . . I am forever whatever I have been at any time for others – and I may at any time be called upon to answer for it – no matter how changed I may be now . . . The self inhabits a character whose unity is given as the unity of a character. (p. 216)

I take from this that each of us is the lead actor in the feature film that is our personal life story, and a co-actor in the films of many others. My identity includes the people, places and symbols that are active in the plots and sub-plots of my 'film'. I will appeal to the cultures of the groups involved to know what I need to be in any specific context.

The health-giving power of coherence helps to explain Antonovski's observation that holocaust survivors who were reconciled to their traumatic past were healthier than those who were not.[9] It helps to explain the central importance of sense-making to organisational success.[10] It helps to explain why both horizontal and vertical integration of health care effort are essential aspects of a healthy society. Each of these instances moves towards coherence-as-a-whole.

Positivism, critical theory, constructivism and a meaningful whole life story are necessary intellectual devices to protect a sense of self

Each person needs to retain a sense that they are a whole integrated self for one obvious reason – without it their sense of self fragments. Quite simply, they become insane (this happened to Pirsig, described in his classic book *Zen and the Art of Motor-cycle Maintenance*. His attempts to describe a philosophy that resolved duality led to a further duality rather than integration – when he realised this he went mad).

The fundamental need to retain the integrity of a sense of self offers an explanation for the three fundamental theories of knowledge I analysed in Chapter 11.

- Whenever I am aware of myself as a discrete entity I give this entity a name to mark its significance – 'me'. I retain the integrity of 'me' by claiming a linear continuity of 'me-ness'. This requires me to assume the mental model of linear thinking. I thereafter will recognise the truth of simple linear direction and compartmentalised identity, which are the assumptions of positivism.
- Being aware of 'me' necessarily brings with it awareness that there are things that are 'not-me'. Here, we find the critical theory mental model of multiple hidden unknowns that may enhance or threaten my sense of self.
- If my sense of self is to evolve, I have to engage with these unknown factors and create from them things that feel part of my identity – my nest of beliefs and web of relationships. Here, we find the insight of constructivism – looking at things 'laterally' to see, or create new connections.
- The result is a life journey that I retrospectively describe as a meaningful story in which I explain how the complex twists and turns experienced along the way make sense as a whole.

If this is correct, these four constructs are necessary consequences of having a conscious identity. We can expect to find them in all aspects of human thought.

Selfishness (that prevents integrating activities) can be seen as a mechanism to protect personal sanity. We do not want to do away with it. We cannot do away with it. What we can do is promote 'enlightened self-interest' – appreciating that mutual inter-dependence is an inescapable reality and valuing others is the same thing as valuing ourselves.

Finding win–win

Enlightened self-interest searches for, and creates win–win.

'Win–win' is a term from transactional analysis, which analyses interpersonal interactions, using the language of 'parent–adult–child'.[11] It reminds us that relationships are developed through games – ideally games in which all sides win. The linear/systemic conflict I repeatedly refer to is a lose–lose game – linear thinking needs whole-system thinking but destroys it; whole-system thinking needs linear focus but damages itself in the process. It can be turned into win–win if the value of both is recognised and the players undertake a dance between the two to see big pictures and immediate focus, long-term aims and short-term steps. Facilitating multi-level dance requires the skills of Mary Poppins or Paulo Friere (chapters 4 and 5). They help people to play together and from this to learn how to do things differently. Multiple actors in multiple scenarios can be considered to interact as in a carnival (Chapter 6), having opportunities to dip in and out of each other's rhythms. Maps and timetables help people to move between different groups and join in appropriately (Chapter 6).

Implications for society

This analysis suggests that successful strategy for integrated primary health care provides opportunities for actors from all parts of the system to find win–win accord. Leadership enables participants from different backgrounds to do this in 'learning spaces' where they share their stories and find imaginative ways forward together. Leadership also connects various learning spaces and enables participants to move between them, sharing their insights and making their efforts more relevant to each other.

The need for win–win explains the importance of the three pillars of primary health care. 'Participation' is the means whereby people can explore and share each other's stories. 'Inter-sectoral collaboration' legitimates collaborative thinking and shared projects. 'Equity' is the value that allows different people to explore new directions as equals without any one player overly dominating others. All aspects of society can work with these principles.

It suggests that health care workers have as part of their role a requirement to help citizens to make meaningful (win–win) connections between different aspects of their health. They can develop a consultation approach that facilitates the unfolding of life stories,[12] and develop team-working that facilitates continuity of care.[13]

It suggests that leaders of organisational change should encourage win–win connections between the insights of staff and the needs of the organisation. Suggestions boxes, think-tanks, consultations, whole-system events and pilot projects can help this.

It suggests that leaders of inter-organisational collaboration need to support sets of teams to connect the organisations that wish to collaborate. These can provide an infrastructure of shared leadership and communication from which shared projects can emerge. Centres to develop shared leadership and explore complex interface issues can do this.

It suggests that PCOs may find theories of whole-system learning and change helpful when considering their policy to integrate primary health care. PCOs can broker academic/practitioner partnerships to promote this.

References

1 Boorse C (1975) On the distinction between disease and illness. *Philosophy and Public Affairs.* **5**: 49–68.
2 Seedhouse D (1989) *Health, the Foundations for Achievement.* John Wiley & Sons, Tiptree.
3 Capra F (2003) *The Hidden Connections.* Flamingo, St Ives.
4 Hanfling O (1987) *Life and Meaning – A Reader.* Blackwell, Pastow.

5 Shotter J (2000) *Conversational Realities – Constructing Life through Language*. Sage, London.

6 Taylor C (1989) *Sources of the Self – The Making of the Modern Identity*. Arcata Graphics, Fairfield, CT.

7 Pertti A (1995) *Researching Culture. Qualitative Method and Cultural Studies*. Sage, London.

8 MacIntyre A (2000) *After Virtue*. Duckworth, London.

9 Antonovsky A (1980) *Health, Stress, and Coping*. Jossey Bass, San Francisco, CA.

10 Weick KE (1995) *Sensemaking in Organizations*. Sage, Thousand Oaks, CA.

11 Berne E (1964) *Games People Play*. Penguin, London.

12 Launer J (1996) You're the doctor, Doctor!: is social constructionism a helpful stance in general practice consultations? *Journal of Family Therapy*. **18**: 255–67.

13 Freeman G and Hjortdahl P (1997) What future for continuity of care in general practice. *BMJ*. **314**: 1870–3.

Chapter 13

Reconciling linear and systems thinking

Summary

In this chapter I consider learning and change in the light of the ideas of the preceding chapters. I draw on the idea of a 'learning organisation' that requires three different types of learning. 'Single-loop learning' involves the accumulation of facts, detection of errors and an approach to change that is incremental. 'Double-loop learning' involves the exploration of new ways of thinking and behaving, and an approach to change that encourages new ways to do things. 'Deutero-learning' involves dynamic interactions between different experiences and ideas to generate new insights about how different things can connect. The concepts of 'learning organisation', 'learning community' and 'incremental revolution' help to develop strategy for ongoing whole system learning and change. In this chapter I also draw conclusions about how to practically apply the ideas presented in this book to develop an infrastructure of leadership for integrated primary health care.

I was having a sea bath on Surprise Beach, enjoying the silky, warm Caribbean water. It was called Surprise Beach because one day the inhabitants of the rickety seashore shacks woke to find that the pebbled beach had changed into a stretch of luxurious sand – the sandy cliff had fallen into a local river and swept the sand to a new purpose.

Surprise and dance are strong in my memory of those carnival days of February 1996. Dominica, the 'Nature Island', is famous for its lush green interior. I had turned up in the little village of St Joseph to meet a friend who did not arrive. I turned to go, but stopped to chat with some locals. We laughed. Music played. We danced. I stayed. I later developed a set of friendships that I could not have imagined at the beginning.

Surprise is created by dance only when the dancers are prepared to adapt to the steps made by the other, creating new shared moves and rhythms. When surprise presents, dance is a good way to respond – by dancing with it rather than running away, being prepared to explore its meaning and potential, neither dominating it nor being dominated by it. I danced verbally with the people I initially met. We joked and laughed, and that gave rise to an initial invitation to share a drink. I danced with their and my expectations, going backwards and forwards from the main town until someone invited me to room in the village. I danced physically in the streets with my new friends and we learned about each other, told each other stories and played games together.

I am using the word *dance* to mean more than a rehearsed sequence of steps. It is a metaphor for dynamic, appreciative interactions between people who are different. Unexpected things happened because all involved were prepared to adapt their moves to each other.

Dynamic, appreciative interaction is at the heart of creating new ways of thinking and acting. It requires putting aside pre-judgements, and being prepared to explore new interpretations – new ways to play. This involves taking risks – taking a risk to trust others and taking a risk to have new experiences. The risk is that this openness exposes you to harm or rejection by others.

Dancing a creative dance requires *love*. In St Joseph, I experienced love to be a spirit of connectedness, generated through a shared effort to create something good. Love is both the input and the output of a shared creative process. It is the energy that keeps the dance going. It is not property but it can be given and rejected. It cannot be predicted but is always to be found. You can only get it if you give it. Love reminds us that 'leaving your heart' and 'finding yourself' are two aspects of the same process of creating something good with others. When this thing has been created, the relationships and the story of the creation become part of the truth of who you are.

As with all phenomena that find expression within dynamic interactions, love is difficult to describe in words – it comes before, and goes beyond words. You know it as a visceral and meaningful experience. Only later do you find words to describe it, to mark it as significant. But these words are thin representations of the experience itself. Humour, dance, belonging, relationships and love all share the property of existing only within the process of dynamic interaction. None fit onto a bar graph. They do not have objective standards that can be measured.

I would have stayed if I knew then of another surprise that awaiting me – the post in South Africa I was heading towards had fallen through. Within two weeks I was to land on the streets of London, homeless and jobless.

Facilitating for surprise

Argyris and Schon highlight the connection between surprise and learning. They write:[1]

> Within the process of inquiry, we give special importance to the experience of surprise, the mismatch of outcome to expectation, which we see as essential to the process by which people can come to see, think and act in new ways. (p. xxiii)

They were writing this as a preface to a book on organisational learning. They reviewed the literature of organisational learning and divided it into practitioner-originated literature of the 'learning organisation' and academic-originated literature of 'organisational learning'. They conclude that authors of the former 'tend to assume, uncritically, that such capabilities [drawing valid inferences from experience] can be activated through the appropriate enablers'. Authors of the latter 'tend to treat observed impediments as unalterable facts of organizational life'. They conclude that both sets of literature underestimate the 'characteristics of behavioral worlds that may inhibit or encourage valid inquiry'.

Argyris and Schon maintain that a theory of organisational learning is possible and important, but much more difficult than it seems at first sight. They offer a 'theory of action perspective' or 'action science' to gain a more realistic insight into how organisations learn and change. This recognises that people have deeply held theories-in-use that obstruct or enable learning and change. These real reasons for people's behaviour are hidden *and* 'undiscussable'.

The end result is that significant learning and innovation happen through a 'fudge' – through mechanisms that bear little relation to the explanations offered.

One example of a fudge is the common metaphor for change: 'carrot and stick'. This is concerned with moving donkeys a short distance. The metaphor gives little insight into sustainable change led by creative, empowered human teams, yet it is commonly used as a meaningful description of what leaders do to cause change.

Another fudge is describing the role of a general practitioner (GP) as a curer of disease. This metaphor gives little insight into how we help people to be whole and healthy, yet it is commonly used as a meaningful description of what we do.

In both cases the 'fudge' is the phenomenon I describe in Chapter 1, whereby the real ideas and motivations that guide behaviour are hidden. These deeply held beliefs about how the world works, and how to relate to it are often hidden even from the individuals themselves. The words they use to explain things can be subconsciously chosen merely to avoid looking at the real issues. A fuller truth is uncomfortable – it might expose inconsistencies or give rise to disagreements with the dominant culture. Exposing these might make you unpopular. You might be marginalised. It can threaten the integrity of your sense of self.

One question for leadership in primary care is whether this matters. As long as things are moving in a good direction, does it matter that the theories of change are inadequate? It does, because leadership cannot be taught without an adequate theory of what is really going on. And holistic practice will die if health workers have to describe their work merely as the cure of diseases. A wrong theory will provoke the wrong actions. Take the example of surprise – it is commonly seen as a failure of leadership in health care not to have anticipated surprises. Yet Argyris and Schon suggest that dealing well with surprise may be a signal success factor. Leadership may need to facilitate its emergence and welcome it as a gift, rather than try to control or deny it.

Three dimensions of learning in learning organisations

Argyris and Schon describe three distinct types of learning needed for a whole organisation to learn: single-loop, double-loop and deutero-learning. They bear close resemblance to the mental models of 'positivism', 'critical theory' and 'constructivism' that I describe in Chapter 11. In Chapter 12 I suggest that these are three fundamental constructs that arise from the ways in which our minds construct ideas.

- Single-loop learning like positivism leaves the underlying assumptions of the status quo intact, and is concerned with detecting error, accumulating facts and incremental change. Single-loop learning is 'linear' thinking – the loop goes back to same place from which it came. It is learning within a controlled laboratory. It is good at examining the status quo and achieving short-term goals.
- Double-loop learning, like critical theory, questions these assumptions and examines deeper, hidden or more complex factors that contribute to the way things are, and might become. Double-loop learning actively looks outside of

the laboratory for hidden mental models and novel interpretations – the loops end up in other places.

* Deutero-learning, includes processes of 'learning how to learn', which, like constructivism, require creative dynamic interaction between different people and ideas.

If single-loop learning asks 'What is on the table?', double-loop learning might ask 'What alternatives are there to tables?' And deutero-learning creates new options to consider.

Argyris and Schon attribute the concept of deutero-learning to Bateson.[2] It is a domain of dynamic interaction between different things, from which comes new and imaginative ideas. This domain is of particular significance in this book because it is the means whereby two different life stories become relevant to each other – the magic that builds a relationship. It is the essential process that integrates diverse activities. It is the exploratory dance to create new rhythms. It is the process of reflecting one idea against others to find new ways of bringing together different worlds of understanding.

When new connections are found they are experienced as a 'gestalt', when parts become connected as a meaningful whole. This moment is the lateral thinking of a comedian who makes a funny association between different ideas. It is the 'flash of recognition', the 'spirit of understanding', when 'the penny drops'.

Bateson describes this process as 'learning-how-to-learn'. This exploratory, connecting process is 'fractal' as explained in complexity theory – predictably present but never tangible. If you try to grasp it you lose it. Bateson writes about deutero-learning:[2]

> the subject has acquired a habit of looking for contexts and sequences of one type rather than another, a habit of 'punctuating' the stream of events to give repetitions of a certain type of meaningful sequence. (p. 166)

This is 'pattern recognition'. It is what a couple does to make their different interests enhancing of each other, what a health professional does to understand what a patient is really saying, what a multi-disciplinary team does to make their collective effort more than the sum of the parts.

In each instance one person reaches out to unknown others to find new ways to play. This is neither the property of one nor the other. It is the moment of co-creation.

Surfacing mental models provokes defensive behaviour

Argyris and Schon make the observation (p. 281) that most organisational 'fixes' or reforms are single-loop, even when undertaken by those who espouse double-loop learning. Furthermore, they claim the extraordinary fact that most reforms are 'subverted by a generic defensive pattern that undermines both single-loop learning and double-loop learning'. They argue that this is because the real motivations and ways of thinking are hidden. They suggest that surfacing them is the antidote to this.

They continue this theme in an essay designed to distinguish action science from participatory action research.[3] The difference in their view is that action science 'places a central emphasis on the spontaneous, tacit theories-in-use that participants bring to practice and research, especially whenever feelings of embarrassment or threat come into play.'

By contrast, participatory action research emphasises that 'some of the people in the organisation or community under study participate actively with the professional researcher throughout the research process from the initial design to the final presentation of results and discussion of their action implications'.[4] (p. 20)

They continue: 'We want to emphasize, however that we see action science and participatory action research as members of the same action research family . . . [that] are aligned in a basic and consequential conflict with normal social science. What they have in common far outweigh their differences.'

This 'basic conflict with normal science' resonates with my observation that those who think mainly in linear ways respond defensively to successful whole-system interventions (Chapter 1). Whole-system change, like participatory action research and action science, invites people who have different insights and understandings to agree a shared long-term vision and what new insights will help them to decide steps towards this. The process challenges all involved to modify their understandings to fit better with those of others. This notion of ongoing mutual adaptation is in basic conflict with the ideas of normal science that promote the idea of unchanging objective reality.

Action science, in particular, requires inner reflection to check if what someone says is what he or she really means. Whole-system change in particular presents people with what they said they wanted, perhaps to find that this conflicts with their hidden inner motivations. In different ways they expose internal/external inconsistencies.

The problem comes when the exposure of inconsistency threatens something important in the identity of an individual or group. This can feel like a fragmentation of their whole sense of self – something to be fiercely resisted.

Here is a catch. On one hand, people want internal/external coherence in order to enhance their sense of self (Chapter 12). On the other, the route to achieving this *co*herence involves recognising and addressing their own *inco*herence. What they thought was a simple well-controlled intervention for change becomes a journey of inner transformation that leaves them feeling confused. In defence they externalise this internal confusion onto others.

The prevalence of strong reactions to exposing internal/external inconsistencies questions the safety of acting on Argyris and Schon's conclusion that hidden theories-in-use should be surfaced – people can get hurt. Furthermore, the argument of Chapter 12 suggests that surfacing them must produce win–win ways forwards if any good is to come from it. Without this someone may feel trapped in a corner from which there is no face-saving exit.

If this was an isolated phenomenon it may not matter. After all, everyone should be allowed some inconsistency. However, as Argyris and Schon point out, most reforms are subverted by this phenomenon of people hiding their true motivations and ways of thinking. People habitually create diversions to avoid looking at the things that matter. This is not an isolated phenomenon.

Locating linear thinking inside whole-system thinking

Here, again, is the lose–lose clash of linear and systems thinking. The changes that people say they want seem at first sight to be straightforward. But in reality they are complex. Externally it requires synchronous change in those things that are dependent on each other. Internally it requires looking at one's own inner world and rectifying inconsistencies. Each person has to listen – really listen – to what he or she is himself or herself saying. It requires listening – really listening – to what others are saying and trying to see things through their eyes. It requires rising to the challenge of the unforeseen consequences of change. Many find this too painful. It is easier to lament the 'impossibility' of change than to engage with the challenges it makes. Many continue to speak empty words.

Let me recapitulate the places where this lose–lose dynamic appears.

- In Chapter 9 I describe the WHO experience that comprehensive primary health needs focused targets – in turn these produce hierarchical infrastructure that works against comprehensive primary health care.
- In Chapter 10 I describe how inability to describe the art and mystery of general practice results in it being defined solely in terms of disease management – in turn this threatens to destroy the role of general practice.
- In Chapter 11 I describe how distrust of qualitative and participatory approaches to enquiry has resulted in them being considered subordinate to quantitative approaches – yet they are means by which the best quantitative focus is found.
- In Chapter 12 I describe how doing practical things to improve health diverts attention away from developing a whole integrated person – which in turn reduces their overall health.

One problem is that many people assume that one way of thinking (linear or systems) must 'drive' the other, or is more fundamental or important than the other. My belief is different (Chapter 11) – these theories/paradigms/mental models are different lenses with which to view a world that is more complex than any lens can ever reveal. They are fundamental theories that arise from the ways in which our minds construct ideas. They are equal but different (Chapter 12).

There is room for linear thinking inside systems thinking if it is considering a part inside a whole. Systems thinking can accommodate the idea that ongoing movement between parts and wholes creates and affirms both. But the linear construct cannot accommodate non-linear thinking – you cannot fit a whole inside a part.

This points to a possible way to turn lose–lose into win–win. Society could value systems thinking above linear thinking and demand ongoing movement between the two. In this case leadership as sense-making would take precedence over leadership as heroic individual acts; health as meaningful stories would take precedence over disease categories; whole-system change would take precedence over simple projects; contextual evolving stories would take precedence over discrete scientific evidence. Leaders would be judged by the degree to which they use discrete focused activity (e.g. curing diseases) to illuminate the more integrated idea (health).

Leadership as sense-making would include the responsibility to help people to become epistemologically aware, able to equally value discrete and inter-connected truths and facilitate reflection on both subjective and objective interpretations. Leaders know that this can be an uncomfortable process that will surface inconsistencies between what people say and what they mean. They know that the process involves some kind of inner transformation as well as external system transformation, and this can be painful and confusing. But they also know that it can be liberating, helping people to both find themselves and leave their hearts inside an evolving story. So how can this be practically achieved?

From whole-system transformation to multiple incremental revolutions

McNulty and Ferlie evaluated a whole-system intervention to transform Leicester Royal Infirmary (LRI) between 1992 and 1997.[5] This hospital was chosen because 'the underlying organizational conditions were seen as positive: if process redesign could work anywhere in the health sector, it would be here' (p. 74).

Based on 'business process re-engineering' the intervention was intended to facilitate a 'big bang' radical transformation of the whole institution towards systems and process thinking. It involved: 'delayering of bureaucracy and top-down hierarchies as departmental structures are dismantled and replaced by process teams' (p. 24); it was 'objective and outcome focused, a fresh start, holistic; radical and rapid; driven from the top down using a process team infrastructure' (p. 26). It had sustained and charismatic top management support – 'top-led but bottom-fed' – and involved multiple parallel redesign projects that helped to 're-envision[ing] the company and invent[ing] new ways of doing things' (p. 30). It was intended to cause 'sharp and simultaneous shifts in strategy, distribution of organisational power, structure and control mechanisms' (p. 32). This approach to change recognises all members of an organisation are 'in a web of values, norms beliefs, taken-for-granted assumptions, that are partially of their own making' (p. 36) and consequently makes sure that: 'leading change is seen as involving action by people at every level of the organisation' (p. 40).

From August 1994 management consultants were appointed as external change agents to work with internal change agents who were seconded from their existing roles (p. 125). They planned to re-engineer six core processes within the hospital in sequence starting with patient visit and patient test. In March 1995 they changed this plan to include concurrent redesign of the four core processes of 'emergency entry', 'patient stay', 'patient visit' and 'clinical support services'. Thirty LRI staff members were involved in four re-engineering laboratories and 50–70 re-engineering projects spanned a wide breadth of clinical directorates, departments and specialities (p. 126). In November 1995 the number of re-engineering projects swelled to over 100 (p. 128).

However, the intervention did not have the desired affect of transforming the culture from bureaucratic to systemic functioning. When the team of external consultants withdrew, the redesign teams and committees largely dissolved and the organisational structures more or less reverted to what they were at the outset. The language of re-engineering almost disappeared from the staff at LRI, and was replaced by the language of 'incremental revolution' (p. 129).

There were nevertheless many successes in discrete areas, and these were particularly likely to happen when there was good practitioner/manager collaboration (p. 359), and when there was synchrony between management and clinical agendas (p. 270).

I am interested in this case study because it aimed for whole-system learning and change, through whole-system ownership – ideas I advocate. However, I am also not surprised that it did not achieve its ambitions because it imagined transformation to be possible in one place – a hospital – in isolation from other actors in the whole system. Reviewing the case reminds me of the following things that I have learned and that I have covered in this book.

- The territory is difficult both theoretically and practically – the LRI project was intensive and expensive, led by skilled people who knew the literature, in an organisation ready for change – and it still didn't work.
- Changing the way people think and behave is a long-term goal. They have to change their cherished and fundamental ideas and this takes time. 'Big bang' interventions are only the beginning of ongoing sustainable change. Sequential cohorts of multi-disciplinary teams are needed to lead projects that are relevant to the needs of the moment and meaningful to the longer-term story. Whole-system change requires ongoing senior management support and long-term investment in infrastructure that supports continual reflection, action and co-adaptation.
- Success comes from synchrony between different motivations for change – shared leadership facilitates multi-disciplinary practitioner/manager, practitioner/academic and generalist/specialist partnerships. Simultaneous and complementary change is needed in all parts of a whole system (in a hospital for example this includes all stakeholders in the multiple care pathways that involve hospital practitioners).
- Improving health is far more complex and contextual than selling products – the application of organisational change methods from the business sector may be misguided. For example, it may be unhelpful to reduce professional autonomy, compared with investing in teambuilding and systems awareness.

The approach I am advocating builds from these four reminders by exhorting the following.

- All who care about sustainable quality improvements in health care need to learn how to think about whole systems and how to work effectively with them.
- A long-term strategy is needed that facilitates incremental revolutions en route to whole system transformation; stakeholders must evaluate a breadth of short- and long-term goals, and set short bursts of innovation within a bigger picture of change.
- Health care needs an infrastructure of multi-disciplinary facilitation and communication that spans organisations, disciplines and geographic areas, and understands how to facilitate meaningful interaction between people and diverse perspectives that facilitates organic whole-system development.
- A fuller vision for health is needed that moves beyond health as a commodity. The appropriateness of models of change derived in business to this bigger vision should be re-evaluated.

'Incremental revolution' can be compared to a boat that goes to sea on a long voyage. When a plank leaks the sailors replace it with another – and another, and another . . . An entirely new boat comes back with everything changed. The sailors never felt affronted by the changes. They did it themselves, when they were ready, and the rationale for each new plank was clear.

But the sailors do not make an exact replica of the original plank. They use whatever resources they have to deal with the leak, mindful of their vision for the potential of the whole journey. This vision changes as they are affected by the cultures, technologies and ideas they experience in the various places they visit. At any point in the voyage they strive to use both external and internal resources to move towards their evolving vision.

From incremental revolutions to ongoing whole-system transformation

Leaders can better apply external resources to their situation when they have a breadth of experience to decide what might work. Sailors who have new ideas about possible destinations and deeper insight into the skill of their crew will alter their views about where they are going and what kind of boat will get them there. They will use the opportunity of a leak to change the boat incrementally to make it better fit for this purpose.

So, too, in organisations, people will adopt external innovations when they help move forward their organisational mission. Leaders match external resources and knowledge with internal shared vision, individual motivations and 'absorptive capacity' ('incorporating the organization's existing knowledge base, 'learning organization' values and goals, technological infrastructure, leadership and knowledge sharing, and effective boundary-spanning roles with other organizations').[6]

Greenhalgh and co-researchers provide a synthesis of the literature of innovation diffusion in service organisations.[6] She notes how contemporary literature recognises that the adoption of an idea from other places relates to its perceived relevance to a 'user system'. A cork may be an ideal cure for a leak caused by a small hole, but not for a rotten set of planks. A map of the world is useful for a boat intended to circle the globe, but not for one about to be decommissioned. In their language my boats are 'user systems'.

In each 'user system' people share an identity of being 'boat-members'. All take part in an adventure that will evolve their personal life stories as well as their shared story. Different people in different user systems will make different decisions about which external ideas to adopt, or adapt to their own internal ideas, depending on where they are in their stories.

Sustainable development of integrated primary health care

The idea of multiple user systems undertaking journeys helps to conceptualise what organisational support is needed for sustainable development of integrated primary health care. As well as recognising the dynamic interaction between internal and external contexts, we must expect multiple user systems to undergo learning and change in response to their evolving vision, leaks that have to be repaired, what new worlds of understanding they encounter, and the different kinds of interactions they have with other user systems.

A common situation is for this natural process of co-evolution to cause conflicts as one ideology or cultural group gains dominance to the extent that it marginalises and oppresses others. This results in simplistic polarisations of whole groups as 'right' and 'wrong'. This leads to ghettos, prejudice and silo-mentality. Integrated primary health care requires that diverse user systems remain engaged in an ongoing dance of social evolution in which equity is a shared value. This requires a network of shared social spaces where different people of different user systems can come together in different combinations. It requires that leaders in these spaces develop them as 'learning spaces' where different people feel comfortable to tell their stories and explore their different understandings of the world.

This points to useful policy about organisational support for both horizontal and vertical integration of primary health care.

- Organisations need to create 'learning spaces' where individuals can learn from and with each other to develop and lead shared projects. These spaces must be accessible, in-between as well as within organisations, and of a size where participants feel able to contribute creatively. Hence the importance of shared geographic areas such as localities, and their connection with larger geographic areas such as PCOs and large sectors. Hence the importance of methods such as 'Open Space',[7] which help multiple voices to be heard and valued within large groups that comprise many different traditions and needs.
- It requires an approach to enquiry and change such as 'appreciative enquiry',[8] which establishes what excites and gives meaning to people and what is their shared vision. These frame the development of multiple simultaneous 'incremental revolutions', building shared projects from positive enthusiasm for change.
- It requires that universities, PCOs and professional groups support the development of whole-system, multi-level collaborations, and take complementary roles in a sustainable infrastructure of facilitation and communication.

These will provide the space, the methods and the organisational support needed to facilitate ongoing whole-system conversations intended to keep the multiple stakeholders of primary health care connected.

The theory of Chapter 12 offers an explanation for why it may be a winning strategy to facilitate multiple connected 'incremental revolutions' set inside ongoing whole-system conversations and supported by statutory institutions. Individuals seek coherent life stories and their identities are formed through webs of relationships. If leadership allows substantial parts of the inter-connected webs to stay the same, while pioneers explore other aspects, feeding back intelligence to the whole community, their sense of identity is largely unchanged. Like sailors on a long voyage they are changing a plank. On one hand, this may not feel like an assault on their sense of self. On the other, the exploratory projects may feel like meaningful development of their shared narrative.

This is what happens in a 'learning community' – many co-existing communities share a vision for a healthy society that builds on things they know to be good. Progress towards this vision is made incrementally and opportunistically, each stage prompting a review of the vision in the light of progress made.

Community members systematically develop the disciplines of a learning organ-isation. Ongoing feedback and cross-organisational shared leadership keep the whole boat balanced even in the high seas.

Primary care organisations as learning communities

The term 'learning community' is associated with Etienne Wenger. He argues that the success of organisations depends on their ability to design themselves as 'social learning systems' and participate in broader learning systems, such as an industry, a region, or a consortium.[9]

Wenger maintains that a social learning system includes: 'a social definition of learning in terms of social competence and personal experience, and three distinct modes of belonging through which we participate in social learning systems: engagement, imagination, and alignment'.

PCOs have the structures to achieve this. Large numbers of discrete organ-isations (e.g. hospitals, general practices, unscheduled care services) can be designed as social learning systems. The broader learning system includes the PCOs and partner agencies. 'Social competence' can be improved through team-working and shared leadership. There is an abundance of 'personal experience', and opportunities for more. 'Engagement', 'imagination' and 'alignment' can be worked out horizontally in localities and networks, and vertically through care pathways.

Conclusions

If the idea of a 'learning community' were to be translated into UK primary care it could take the following form.

At an individual level

Practitioners are skilled reflective practitioners, able to use qualitative and participatory as well as quantitative methods of enquiry within the consulting room. They are skilled at listening to themselves and to others – to what they say and also what they really mean. They help others to see their specific complaints in the context of their whole life stories. This practitioner is epistemologically aware and recognises that they are always other ways to look at things, and what you see at first is never the whole story. They are always fishing for surprises, and new insight into what health means to someone.

Aided by computer decision-support, the practitioner knows about local services, care pathways and guidelines. As part of professional life he or she dips in and out of local planning groups and later in their career (when they have become skilled in their health worker role) they rotate through part-time roles in different parts of the system, contributing to shared leadership for various issues, vertically and horizontally.

Different and innovative windows into practitioner performance are valued, including audio and video analysis, peer review, 360° appraisal, knowledge questionnaires, audit and research projects, written papers, significant events, student teaching and facilitating team-learning. These are presented not as defensive posturing, but as a proud celebration of personal growth.

It is an expected part of professional life to step in and out of leadership roles that help colleagues to make sense of the whole system. In different contexts this might be called management, facilitation, mentorship or citizenship.

At an organisational level

Small enterprises (general practices, pharmacists, dentists) use the principles of a 'learning organisation', helping all staff to develop the habit of learning from and with each other, and facilitating 'learning spaces'. Systems and feedback loops help to translate individual learning into whole-organisation learning and change.

PCOs help small enterprises and networks to adopt principles of organisational learning and contribute to shared leadership for local learning and change.

Each organisation names a multi-disciplinary team to lead for quality, including practice-based commissioning, research, audit and organisational development. PCOs support the development of these teams to become increasingly able.

Certain general practices become 'R&D practices' skilled at local leadership for quality, including collaborative research, audit and whole-system learning and change.

Data are gathered both routinely and in response to emerging issues, and fed back to those who generate it so they can learn. They are used to build up a rich picture of the organisations, local communities and the whole sector.

Audits (quantitative, qualitative and participatory) led by multi-disciplinary teams document the development of the organisation. Sequential audits are connected one with another to facilitate a string of incremental changes which, over time, engage all staff in initiatives that facilitate ongoing adaptation of the whole organisation.

Management encourages imaginative and ethical experiments within agreed groundrules, ensuring competent evaluation, good project management and timely feedback.

At the level of the locality

PCOs support localities as 'cells' that enable internal innovation and external connections. Leaders are charged with integrating efforts for health both horizontally where they develop cross-organisation collaborations, and vertically where they develop care pathways. Those who are skilled at community development, for example the voluntary sector, schools and churches, help think through practical ways to engage people and connect diverse efforts.

Whole-system events enable stakeholders from all parts of the system to revisit their shared vision and develop multi-disciplinary teams to explore issues of the moment. System maps make transparent how to navigate the whole system. Feedback loops ensure that learning at one stage fuels later learning.

Initiatives promote win–win collaborations, for example Timebank (which enables people to gain community credits), 'one-stop shops' (which signpost an array of services) and arts programmes (which encourage creative interaction).

Centres support leadership development. Here, leaders from different disciplines learn from and with each other, plan integrated services and support things that help people to visualise individual journeys through complexity, such as patient-held records and 'how to understand the system' booklets.

Networks connect need and enthusiasm. They cross organisational boundaries and connect enthusiasts for audit, research and action for change. Networks of networks help broker coalitions of interest for a diversity of constituencies.

Consortia of partner organisations support shared leadership and collaborative enquiries, creating pathways between research, audit and clinical effectiveness. They co-ordinate 'whole-system participatory action research', which includes quantitative, qualitative and participatory enquiries. Multi-disciplinary teams of leaders support action learning. Innovation is showcased locally and in other areas.

R&D systems help academic/practitioner partnerships to develop research and audit projects in response to local need. Data gathered from GP computer systems and other sources are amalgamated and fed back to stakeholders so they can learn.

New projects build from previous learning, lever in other resources and contribute to sustainable infrastructure for ongoing whole-system learning and change.

Formative training

In addition to the specific competencies required of different roles, all health care practitioners learn how to work with whole systems. They are trained to be epistemologically aware, understanding the contextual nature of knowledge and the value of complementary theories of knowledge. They use a broad concept of health, recognising that each contributes only a part to overall health, and that their own work is enhanced by the contributions of others.

Trainee health workers experience the evolving nature of the 'real world' by revisiting the same locality year after year where they become temporary members of teams developing and questioning these issues. Here they can also learn team skills and evaluate care pathways.

Spirals of learning that connect personal, organisational and service development are modelled throughout undergraduate courses. Ability to conduct personal and collaborative enquiries that result in change is learnt at an early stage and revisited at increasing levels of complexity throughout training. Horizontal and vertical integration of care is illuminated through team projects. Ability to map different contributions to overall health is learnt by exercises that demonstrate the complementary value of a range of contributions to a healthy society, including public health, environmental health and community health.

Leadership style

Leadership recognises that at every level and every stage participants may find the processes of organisational learning personally confronting, feeling like an unwelcome and risky exploration of uncertainty. Safe learning environments – 'learning spaces' – at all levels of the system help them to explore difficult things. Skilled facilitation and leadership makes things seem fun, easy and instantly rewarding. Boundaries are chosen to stretch people, but not so far as to break them.

Shared leadership between different organisations, portfolios and disciplines supports inter-organisational innovation and aligns communication systems. System maps, nodes and whole-system events connect their networks.

Leadership helps people to make sense of complex situations by clarifying what is known, legitimising doubt and encouraging enquiry and innovation. They model the pillars of comprehensive primary health care, and the disciplines of a learning organisation. They encourage life-long learning and enquiry in which personal, service and organisational development are intertwined. They encourage descriptions of contexts, narratives, multiple perspectives, multiple approaches to enquiry and a breadth of appropriate data which help to locate specific activities within rich evolving stories.

Leadership happens at every level and every place, and is not seen as the domain of certain individuals. Leaders clarify what is the specific system of concern so people can focus on practical realities rather than theoretical ideas. The academic level of leadership programmes relates less to the knowledge content and more to the complexity of change being led.

Leadership initiatives include short bursts of action within a longer-term shared vision for health. These draw on the principles of participatory action research, action science and action learning to ensure that participants reflect on the issues that really matter to them. Participants use their daily work as case studies for learning. Three cycles of reflection and enquiry are connected to encourage incremental progress that leads to more substantial longer-term evolution.

Providing the organisational support for these would be the responsibility of many different organisations.

- PCOs provide the funding and political support for leadership development and real-life experience with which to reflect and listen, and test out new ideas. They develop cross-portfolio team-working to counter the tendency of bureaucratic structures to stifle innovation.
- General practices and other community organisations provide an interface between medical and non-medical aspects of health. Some practitioners develop portfolio careers to help counter a tendency towards professional insularity.
- Networks of networks enable multiple organisations and stakeholders to form coalitions of interest and shared leadership for a variety of issues.
- Cross-sectoral consortia provide authority and pathways for research, audit, organisational development and leadership. They relate to development support centres to help counter a tendency to consider only statutory needs.
- Professional bodies encourage members to argue what quality practice requires and its specific local application. They develop multi-disciplinary platforms for this to help counter a tendency to overly serve uni-disciplinary interests.
- Higher education institutions provide a series of connected programmes of learning in partnership with local health care partners. These include research and audit as mechanisms for learning and change, and multiple methods enquiry with participatory and qualitative aspects. Academic/practitioner partnerships embed audit and research within ongoing cycles of local reflection and action.
- Funding and statutory bodies reward efforts to integrate primary health care. Universities are better rewarded for leading complex interventions, comparative case studies, multiple methods research and academic/practitioner partnerships. PCOs are rewarded for creating pathways between audit and

research, for facilitating whole-system events, and for creating sustainable academic/practitioner/manager leadership that embeds enquiry within a local learning community.

References

1 Argyris C and Schon DA (1996) *Organizational Learning 2 – Theory, Method, and Practice.* Addison Wesley, Reading, MA.
2 Bateson G (2000) *Steps to an Ecology of the Mind.* University of Chicago Press, Chicago, IL.
3 Argyris C and Schon DA (1991) Participatory action research and action science compared. In: WF Whyte (ed) *Participatory Action Research.* Sage, New York, NY.
4 Whyte WF (1991) *Participatory Action Research.* Sage, New York, NY.
5 McNulty T and Ferlie E (2002) *Reengineering Health Care – the Complexities of Organizational Transformation.* Oxford University Press, Oxford.
6 Greenhalgh T, Robert G, Macfarlane F, Bate P and Kyriakidou O (2004) Diffusion of innovations in service organizations: systematic review and recommendations. *The Milbank Quarterly.* **82**: 581–629.
7 Owen H (1997) *Open Space Technology – A User's Guide.* Berrett-Koehler, San Francisco, CA.
8 Whitney D and Trosten-Bloom A (2003) *The Power of Appreciative Inquiry.* Berrett-Koehler, San Francisco, CA.
9 Wenger E (2000) Communities of practice and social learning systems. *Organization.* **7**: 225–46.

Part IV

Techniques that integrate linear and systems thinking

This part describes practical techniques. The facilitation teams I have worked with have found these useful with front-line primary care practitioners and managers, with senior management teams and with large multi-disciplinary groups.

These are prompts, not protocols. I aim to describe why they are useful and what they look like so you can decide whether you want to explore them further. It is up to you to apply them, and develop them, to meet your particular needs.

To develop our skills we often used team reflections at the end of meetings to learn. We found this to be fun and effective. Sometimes one team member would observe another facilitating a meeting and give feedback later. We used external consultants at times and attended courses ourselves, but these became less necessary when we become good at learning from each other.

Remember to claim sufficient authority to intervene in these techniques. For example, in role-play you need prior agreement to step in if people get caught up in damaging interactions. Extra chairs in a group circle allow you to slip in and out with minimal disturbance.

You have a responsibility to give positive energy to the room. This includes modelling good meeting behaviour and appreciating that of others. It means preventing the squashing of someone's off-beat ideas and active listening to tease out ideas. Humour and putting into words what many are thinking can be helpful.

Careful planning is essential. Without this you will be caught out by the simplest of things. In a well-planned meeting you will be 'totally present and absolutely invisible'. Unpleasant conflict rarely happens but if it does this is a time when you need to be as cool as cool, using your personal skills and team members to allow emotions to be acknowledged, responded and melted away. You may at times have to give a sense of invulnerability and confidence, even when you don't feel it inside. You may have to intervene swiftly when you see danger. Timing is important – like a cricket player, hesitation and premature action both catch you out, and good timing can produce a sweetly driven ball to the boundary rope. Remember to smile.

Chapter 14

Mapping the system of concern

Summary

When you have identified a concern, you are likely to think of people, ideas and resources that could help understand and improve it. However, there will be other people, insights and resources that you have not thought of that are needed for a good outcome. To work with these things you must first know what they are. This chapter describes five exercises to identify them.

For each concern you need to frame an aspect of it as a simple question. For example, this might be 'Who are the stakeholders?' or 'What comes into your mind when . . .' or 'What things influence .?'. The exercises can be done alone but are more powerful when done with a trusted team, because different team members will be stimulated to think of new things in response to the ideas of others. Each exercise initially takes 10–30 minutes, but it gains in strength by subsequent review. By leaving your work on show, perhaps on flip-chart paper on your wall, you can reflect on it days, weeks and months later. New and richer ideas often develop through repeatedly checking back on your work. The exercises are:

- brainstorming and rainbowing – listing things in a fast 'storm of the brain', then drawing connections between them
- nominal grouping with sticky squares or magnetic hexagons – clustering things together, and drawing connections between the groups
- force-field analysis – analysis of power and influence in one particular focus
- drawing a complex power diagram – producing a map of how different factors, including people and organisations, affect each other
- drawing your own life-line – a description of what happened when.

Brainstorming and rainbowing

What this is trying to achieve

A 'brainstorm' is literally a storm of the brain – a rain of unordered ideas. It is good at surfacing subconscious associations and it needs to be done fast to stay in a semi-subconscious domain. When there are no more ideas offered you can be fairly sure that the page contains the things that need to be explored for now. You can then start sorting them.

Instructions

- Write the question for the brainstorm at the top of a piece of flip-chart paper, for example 'What would you like the health centre to look like in five years' time?', 'What research ideas would you like to explore?' or 'Who are the stakeholders for this project?'
  Invite the participants to call out their ideas about this question.
- Write down the exact words used by each contributor, without challenge or debate. You can ask someone to rephrase something or offer them another way of saying it. You are not allowed to reinterpret their words without permission, since this will distort meaning and halt the free-thinking process.
- Invite contributions from throughout the room to keep everyone engaged, quickly shutting down those who want to move into debate.
- Continue until there are no more contributions.
- A variation of this method (developed by Peter Sainsbury) is to put a line down the middle of the paper and have half the room brainstorming one idea and the other a similar idea. This reveals the different things participants associate with the two ideas (examples are 'team' and 'committee', and 'research' and 'audit').

When you feel that people have no more to say, move into a second phase, which validates and clusters these ideas – I call this 'rainbowing'.*

- At a fairly brisk pace repeat out loud each written phrase, inviting agreements or disagreements (observe body language as much as words) and invite participants to prepare their ideas about how the different points might be clustered. You will find that most ideas will be quickly agreed and others can be agreed after rewording. Mark separately the points about which participants 'agree to disagree'. Put on a 'parking board' those things that are important but to be dealt with on another day.
- Using different-coloured flip-chart pens, draw lines between ideas that the group recognises to be connected. At its best this stage seems like an animated whole-room dialogue. When one person overly dominates, the sense of ownership by all is weakened.
- Negotiate with the group what name you wish to call each cluster. Write this down in a different colour. If this leads into the next exercise, rewrite the headings on fresh paper.
- In the resulting written report list the original storm of ideas under the new headings. This enables you to track how your conclusions originated in the original brainstorm.

Common mistakes

- Not making the task clear.
- One person or sub-group overly dominating.
- Writing words other than those people actually said.

---

* This term was adopted by Janet Hayes, a hugely insightful and committed woman. Sadly, she died in December 2003.

Nominal grouping with sticky squares or magnetic hexagons

What this is trying to achieve

Nominal grouping/hexagons help to cluster different ideas, and to think through how to connect different clusters. The techniques described here generate the headings from the ideas but if the headings are already agreed it can be done the other way around. In Chapter 6 I describe how this technique can be used with sticky squares (Post-Its) to gain consensus about development priorities for a locality, and research themes for a research network. Hexagons are particularly useful in small groups who wish to find new ways of connecting existing things, and identify new things to be developed (for example, for organisational policy or personal career choices). Here, I shall describe the technique using hexagons. You can buy these (Magnotes) and find case studies, guides and training from www.logovisual.com.

Instructions

- Write the question you are asking somewhere clearly visible, for example 'What am I going to do with the next 10 years of my life?', 'How can I make this idea fit with mainstream development?' or 'How can I pull together these separate areas of my life/work?', 'How can we improve organisational targets for XXX?' or 'Which groups can help us to achieve XXX?'.
- Identify three different kinds of motivating things that can be built from. At a personal level these may be (in the context of the question): 'What am I good at?', 'What do I like to do?', 'What will others pay me for?'. At an organisational level they might be (in the context of the question): 'What strengths do we have?', 'What internal resources do we have that could be made relevant?', 'What external relationships or connections can we possibly build upon?'. Allocate a different colour pen to each of the three domains.
- Brainstorm each of these three categories, writing each new idea on a separate hexagon in the appropriate colour. Continue until you can think of no more.
- Move the hexagons around, fitting tightly together those that are readily connected, and keeping further away those that are unrelated. Do not worry at this stage if it does not seem to make sense – it may take some time before you can see new coherent patterns. You may need to start again with three new questions. The exercise is helping you to examine the heart of your concern, and what things really are relevant to it, especially those things you are unable to see at first sight. If everything seems to fit neatly together straight away you may be focusing on the wrong issue, or artificially connecting things that are really separate.
- Take a photograph of the hexagon board (or the wall on which you have stuck the sticky squares). This will remind you of your learning journey.
- Focus attention on where the three colours come closely together. Ask yourself if these really are strong connections. If so this is likely to be a good place to build next steps. Move them around again and see if they again still come back strongly together.
- Focus attention on where you want things to come together but they won't.

Put a blank hexagon in between them and try different words on it – what thing might create the link you need to make one relevant to the other(s). What colour does this need to be?

- Leave the board visible and keep going back to it to check the strength of your analysis.

Common mistakes

- Inappropriately fitting hexagons together.
- Becoming overly attached to one solution (try taking favourite hexagons off the board).
- Not persevering for long enough (you may need to leave the board on view for months).

Force-field analysis

What this is trying to achieve

A force-field analysis is an exercise in identifying the forces for and against moving in the direction you want. It is good at identifying forces in a discrete focus.

Instructions

- Write the question for the force-field analysis at the top of a piece of flip-chart paper, for example 'What will help/hinder the gaining funds?', 'What will help/hinder this project to succeed?', 'What will help/hinder my success in this field?'.
- Draw a line down the centre of the page. One the left side write factors that will help. On the right side write factors that will hinder. Continue until you can think of no more factors on either side.
- Draw arrows from the factors you have identified into the middle line. Highlight in a different colour the things over which you have control.
- Redraw the diagram to avoid crowding, putting together similar things. Use thick arrows when influences are strong and thin when they are less strong.
- Stand back and look at the overall pattern. How much in your favour does the whole picture look? Are the thicknesses of the arrows right? Are there things on either side that you have missed? What is your conclusion about whether you can move things in the direction you want? What do you need to prioritise in your plans to ensure success?
- Share the diagram with a trusted 'critical friend'. Ask them to challenge your analysis of which way the balance of forces lies, and whether there are other forces that are acting, or could begin to act.
- Keep the diagram safe. It is your analysis at this moment. Later on, review it and see how the balance of power has changed. With hindsight ask yourself: were the forces for and against as you expected? Were the thicknesses of the arrows accurate? What other factors came into play and why? Why did you not see these coming?

Common mistakes

- Stacking all the forces on one side or another, or applying inappropriate thickness to the arrows, in order to subconsciously persuade yourself of a course of action.
- Not knowing enough about the territory to see the multiple forces at play.
- Attributing forces to be more or less under your control than they really are.

Drawing a complex power diagram

What this is trying to achieve

This produces a diagram of how multiple factors affect each other. The Open University Systems Unit (UK) teaches a variety of types of diagramming (http://technology.open.ac.uk). It differs from a force-field analysis by drawing back from one focus of concern to map multiple inter-connected influences, and using the diagram to explore how the overall system can be changed to alter the balance of power.

   The diagram first notes the various relevant factors and how they influence each other. Second, through redrawing the diagram and gaining fresh eyes into its potential, it can help to understand how new feedback loops and interventions can affect things to your advantage. You may need to redraw it many times as you identify more and more complex interactions. You can use it as a team exercise to gain shared understanding of how to be most effective.

Instructions

- Write the thing you are concerned about in the middle of a piece of flip-chart paper, for example 'high teenage pregnancy rates', 'insufficient funds to continue working' or 'the computer not providing correct information'.
- Write down the various factors that affect the concern in a similar way to a force-field analysis. These can be people, organisations or ideas. Draw arrows into the circle from those things that you think reduce the concern (e.g. youth centres, paid income or computer skills). Draw arrows out from the circle to things that make the concern worse (e.g. peer pressure, mortgage or poor data entry).
- Behind the things you have written, write the names of things that influence them. This will produce a mass of names and arrows criss-crossing the page.
- In a second colour circle the individuals or organisations you wish to influence.
- In a third colour circle your own products – the things you have control over and which may be able to influence the behaviour of others on the page. Draw hard or dotted lines from these to other places, indicating different levels of influence.
- Redraw the diagram to avoid crowding, and to open out areas where some creative thinking can be done about increasing the influence of your products on the overall shape to your advantage. Remove your concern to a more peripheral place. Add in new factors and lines to understand better the whole interplay of forces.
- Take the diagram to your stakeholders – either in a group or one at a time.

Invite them to contribute to redrawing and analysing the diagram. At this point you may have an uncomfortable experience of recognising that your stated concern is not the most helpful one, either to you or to them. Bear with the irritation of this – it may be your most important learning from the exercise.

- Redraw as many times as is necessary to produce a diagram that is recognisable by your stakeholders as useful representation of the factors which affect the concern.
- This is your complex power analysis. In the doing of it you will have identified existing and new places where you could strengthen the impact of the things under your control. The next task is to use this diagram to make decisions about new strategy.

Common mistakes

- Over- or underestimating your own power.
- Mistaking encouraging noises from others as power or influence.
- Being unprepared to think differently about the phenomenon of concern.

Drawing your life-line

What this is trying to achieve

A life-line is a technique to understand how you came to be in the situation you find yourself. This may help you to value better the things you have, re-discover the things you have forgotten, and identify new steps that will help the coherence of your life journey as a whole.

It can be done alone or as a group exercise. In groups it can involve large pieces of paper on the wall with dates (see 'Future search' and 'Open space', Chapter 15). Participants are asked to write things that mattered to them at these times, set against other historical events. Discussions reveal how these things influenced the development of everyone (often in different ways).

Here, I am describing the technique when done alone, to help you to get your present situation in the fuller context of your whole life. Start with a big piece of paper – flip-chart size or bigger. Have different coloured pens available. Then draw in any way you like your life from your birth to the present day. Try to remember how it was then, rather than projecting your feelings of this moment into the past. You can do it as a straight line with dates, as a meandering road, a line of peaks and troughs, or any way that works for you. The purpose is for you to gain insight into your whole life journey – there are no rights or wrongs.

Instructions

- Indicate the high and low times.
- Indicate your successes and failures – what are you most proud of? And least?
- Indicate your greatest challenges; did you struggle through? Or not?
- Indicate your loves and hates – the things that define who you are and who you are not.
- Include your family life, your career in paid work, the ups and downs of your health, your sports and hobbies, your progress as a student/learner.

Stand back from your drawing.

- Look carefully at the overall pattern. Note your use of space, colour, symbols. What feelings does the drawing evoke in you? What person do you see? What strengths and weaknesses? Is this really you?
- Indicate aspects from the past that are drawing you back – perhaps unresolved hurts and fears? What patterns are there about why you get into difficult situations?
- Indicate aspects that define your potential, the 'real you'. Is that person still in the present? What things that are important to you are you neglecting?
- Indicate what helped you to learn most about yourself – what was that learning?
- Are there other people in your life-line – are they pulling you forwards or backwards? What are you doing to them – are you drawing them forwards or backwards?
- Write down quickly on another paper, before you become overly cerebral about it, what you think this is telling you about your next steps?

Common mistakes

- Drawing the diagram as a description only of how you feel at present.
- Overly focusing on optimistic or pessimistic aspects.
- Projecting – drawing people other than yourself.

Chapter 15

Whole-system events

Summary

Sooner or later you will want to bring large numbers of people together to exchange their understandings of a concern, and to find creative new ways forward that are agreed by all. You will already be familiar with some models of large-group events – conferences and carnivals, for example.

A whole-system event is a conference where large numbers of people learn together and move the whole story along. It 'gets the whole system in the room'. It should not be seen as a stand-alone event. Instead, it is one of a series of connected events which help to unfold integrated efforts to improve the whole system.

It requires mechanisms to describe the story, and for participants to move between small and large groups and between different stakeholder groups. It requires opportunities for people to self-organise.

It requires detailed planning and skilled facilitation. The principles of Chapter 5 and the techniques of Chapter 16 will help you to devise your own whole-system event.

In this chapter I describe 'Future search conference' and 'Open space technology' – two well-established models of whole-system events. I quote extracts from the books that describe them. If you intend to try these models out I suggest you read the full accounts, and seek advice from those who have experience of facilitating them.

'Appreciative enquiry' is another very useful approach which adopts the same constructivist principle of creating the future from what is positive about the present (rather than solving problems or reacting to hostility). It involves a cycle of: appreciating what is; imagining what might be; determining what should be; and creating what will be. A good introduction is given in *The Power of Appreciative Inquiry*.[1] You can read about other whole-system methods, including real-time strategic change in *Large Group Interventions – Engaging the Whole System for Rapid Change*. See also the examples in Chapter 4.

'Future search' helps a diverse group of people to explore their past, present and desired future, as a back-drop to co-ordinated action planning. You can read about this in *Future Search – An Action Guide to Finding Common Ground in Organizations and Communities*.[3]

'Open space' enables self-organising groups to deal with complex overlapping issues and develop sets of co-ordinated action plans. You can read about this in *Open Space Technology – A User's Guide*.[4]

I have had the opportunity of being a participant in events of these designs and found them to be effective and enjoyable. I have also enjoyed applying similar principles in much smaller events and training courses. Even dinner parties and team meetings can be whole-system events of a sort, if you want them to be.

So please don't think of these as beyond your reach. The task does become more complex as the diversity and number of stakeholders increases. But it is misunderstandings and previous hurts between participants that cause conflict and failure, and this can happen in small groups as much as in large. I suggest you practise the skills in safe, modest situations.

Future search conference

'Future search' is useful for stakeholders to discover shared intentions, to create a shared future vision for their organisation or community, and to implement a shared vision. For example it could be used to develop collaboration for a new health centre, locality planning, or PCT-led initiatives for integrated services. Sixty to seventy participants are optimal.

The sponsor leads the planning team and this takes some time, including creating a cross-stakeholder planning group and careful targeting of potential participants. Wiesbord and Janoff[3] describe eight conditions for success:

- 'whole-system' in the room
- whole 'elephant' as context for local action
- common ground and future focus, not problems and conflicts
- self-managed small groups
- full attendance
- healthy meeting conditions
- three-day event (sleep twice)
- public responsibility for follow-up.

In the three days participants: review the past; explore the present; create ideal future scenarios; identify common ground; and make action plans (p. 6).

In the first afternoon participants map their memories on a wall of paper. It takes about two and a half hours. Long strips of paper line the walls with titles: 'personal', 'global' and 'X' (the conference focus) (p. 18), with dates every five to ten years. Participants note their own milestones on the paper, then in mixed small groups around flip-charts they discuss the trends and patterns they detect.

The second task uses Buzan's idea of a 'mindmap'[5] to explore the external trends that are having an impact on the conference topic (p. 88). Participants are asked to 'come on down' to the paper. Someone describes a trend, such as 'increased environmental awareness' and the diagrammer draws this as a line out of a central circle that contains the conference focus. A concrete example is written beside the line. For each new idea the group considers if it is a branch from a previous idea or something new. As more and more ideas are put forward different clusters of ideas are marked in different colours.

Before people break at the end of the first day they post seven sticky dots on the trends they consider most important for the conference. These are coloured by stakeholder groups to indicate which groups care most about which trends. Unfinished tasks or issues are acknowledged before finishing for the day.

On day two participants have a close look at the wall and have an open discussion about it, before breaking into stakeholder groups to draw their own version of the mindmap. This clarifies for them what they are most concerned about. In these stakeholder groups they also undergo an exercise in 'prouds and sorrys' – what things has their stakeholding group done that they are proud of, and sorry about.

Before lunch on the second day the mixed groups of the first day reconvene to explore their shared future hopes. They are invited to put themselves five, ten or 20 years into the future, 'imagining that they have made their dreams come true', and list on flip-charts: (a) concrete examples of what has actually happened; and (b) the major barriers they had to overcome on the way (p. 99). In the afternoon they present these to the whole conference in any way they like – drama, a skit, play, TV, etc.

Each scenario group is then asked to write on three flip-charts:

- Common future – 'what we all agree about' (e.g. value statements and abstractions).
- Potential projects – 'how to get what we want' (e.g. concrete proposals, policies).
- Not agreed – recognising conflicts that have not yet been worked through.

When the lists are finished they pair with another group and merge two sets into one. All lists are posted on the wall and the combined lists are cut into strips – one item on each strip.

On the morning of the third day participants group the strips into themes and discuss whether this is a true reflection of their consensus. The rest of the day is taken up with two rounds of action planning from the consensus, starting with the stakeholder groups. The sponsor has the last word. Cross-organisational planning groups move things forward until the next event.

Open space technology

This method allows hundreds of people to self-organise. It is especially good at moving forwards issues that people from different backgrounds agree to be important, but for which no one has 'the answer', and indeed there are multiple complementary 'answers'. It facilitates different disciplines or organisations to develop simultaneous and complementary projects that move things forward. For example, it would be a good method to generate a diversity of efforts within a town or city to address issues such as care of the elderly or drug abuse.

It can take one to three days: 'In one day the conversations will be stimulating and intense. In two days, that conversation will be recorded for posterity. With three days, priorities can be established and next steps identified'.[4]

Participants first stand in a circle in a 'market place of ideas'. Whoever wishes steps into the middle and describe a discussion group they would like to convene. As many people as want do this: 'Groups of 25–50 have about 30 issues, groups of 100–200 have about 75 issues'.[4] They write their name and the issue on a piece of paper on the 'wall' – the 'community bulletin board'.

Participants buzz around the 'wall', which includes the daily schedule, and the pieces of paper are posted on a 'space/time matrix'. A few sessions become combined and other times changed so they do not coincide, but for the most part the schedule is fixed fairly quickly.

Then everyone goes to the groups of their choice, often about 90 minutes per group session. The convenor writes up notes of the meeting there and then (often using a computer in the main room), with the headings 'Title', 'Convenor', 'List of participants', 'Discussion & Recommendations'. These summaries are posted on the 'wall' and become part of the conference report.

It requires a microphone for the plenary sessions, one break-out room per 20 participants, one flip-chart per breakout room, marker pens, sticky squares and masking tape, and one computer per 20 participants. Refreshments are available continuously.

Owen attributes the success of these events to 'creating time and space, and holding time and space' (p. 57).[4] The facilitator is 'totally present and absolutely invisible'.

The 'rule of two feet' allows people to go wherever they like when they like. 'Bumblebees' constantly flit between one group and another, often cross-pollinating ideas, and 'butterflies' do very little as 'centers of non-action' (p. 100), but somehow cause significant conversations 'perhaps significance emerges precisely because no-one is looking for it'. Owen advocates four signs posted in prominent places (pp 72–3):

The Theme (briefly stated)

The Four Principles:

- Whoever comes is the right people
- Whatever happens is the only thing that could have
- Whenever is starts is the right time
- When it's over, it's over

The One Law:

- The Law of Two Feet

An Exhortation:

'Be prepared to be surprised'

The community assembles twice a day – for morning announcements and evening news. The simple structure and rules provide a space that is flexible and enabling for self-organising and multiple adaptations.

References

1 Whitney D and Trosten-Bloom A (2003) *The Power of Appreciative Inquiry*. Berrett-Koehler, San Francisco, CA.
2 Benedict Bunker B and Aban B (1997) *Engaging the Whole System for Rapid Change*. Jossey-Bass, San Francisco, CA.
3 Weisbord M and Janoff S (2000) *Future Search – An Action Guide to Finding Common Ground in Organizations and Communities*. Berrett-Koehler, San Francisco, CA.
4 Owen H (1997) *Open Space Technology – A User's Guide*. Berrett-Koehler, San Francisco, CA.
5 Buzan T (1976) *Use Both Sides of Your Brain*. Dutton, New York, NY.

Chapter 16

Facilitating learning in groups

Summary

There are ways to run a meeting that make the most of its potential to learn new things from participants, and ways that consolidate previous agreements. Both are needed. There are things you can do to improve the potential of the meetings you lead to do both. This chapter summarises the following techniques.

- Switching between chairing and facilitating a meeting – a chair holds the reins of control to get business done – contributions go back and forth to the chair. A facilitator enables learning by maximising interactions between participants – contributions consequently go around the room, often bypassing the leader. Skilled chairs and facilitators move repeatedly between both modes to keep participants engaged and creative.
- Checklist for a meeting – a list of easy-to-forget things.
- Centering the learning space – the story, energisers, ground rules and evaluation.
- Small-group–large-group iterations – connecting the intimacy of small-group reflections with whole-group consensus.

These techniques all help to provide an environment where individuals constantly reflect their own experiences against bigger, evolving pictures. They prevent people becoming lost either in 'blue-sky thinking' or 'navel gazing'. Instead they help keep people rooted in the practical potential of the moment.

Switching between chairing and facilitating a meeting

Meetings usually need a combination of sharp re-establishment of what is known, and interactive, creative generation of new ideas. The balance depends on the context. But if you have too much 'top down' re-establishment of what is known, people disengage and feel that they are merely rubber-stamping other people's dictates. Conversely, if there is too much 'bottom up' creativity it can feel laborious and time-wasting – 'reinventing wheels'. Switching between 'chairing' and 'facilitating' a meeting can avoid these problems.

The essence of chairing a meeting is that comments go back and forth to that one person. A diagram of interactions between committee members will show that they go 'through the chair'. It is intentionally a linear and controlled process. The consequence is that the 'committee' can feel one-dimensional, formal and stifling.

The essence of facilitating a meeting is that multiple conversations take place between participants. A diagram of interactions between committee members will show that they go in multiple directions that often bypass the chair. It is intentionally a systemic process where ideas spark off ideas in the others. The consequence is that the 'team' experience can be of exciting and fun, noisy and chaotic.

Skilled leaders of meetings constantly switch between one mode and the other to both enable creative participation, and to get the work done. They actively seek contributions from those they know have useful things to say, and those who have been overly quiet for too long.

Interesting discussions may need to be guillotined. A 'parking board' may be needed to mark conversations for another day. New emerging problems may need to be opened out. The leader does not follow a set way of doing things but follows the energy in the room, mindful of the time constraints and the full agenda, wanting to 'keep people on their toes', creative at the cusp between what is known and what is not.

Exercises

- Explain to participants that you are trying to switch between the two modes. Ask them to give feedback about how this helps and hinders.
- Invite a meeting member to draw the lines of interaction in the meeting. Examine this diagram later, either alone or shared with team members or a mentor.
- Video or tape-record the meeting. Play it back to yourself later and write down what you are learning about your personal way of being effective when leading meetings.

Checklist for a meeting

The overall idea

- Write down exactly what is the purpose of the meeting and what is your budget?
- Brainstorm who are the right people to attend and map the system of concern.
- What levers do you have to get the people you want there?

The timing

- Is it happening when it will fit with other needs (e.g. new policy or end of year reports)?
- Is it happening at a place and time that your target group can attend?
- Have you advertised in the best way, and given them enough notice to attend?

Planning the programme

- Write down the learning objectives of the meeting and the intended outputs.
- Use backwards mapping to identify what needs to happen at each stage of the meeting.
- Write the meeting programme, making sure there is enough participation.

Planning the format

- What mix of knowledge – expert speaker/leaders of projects/participant-generated?
- How will small-group–large-group iteration lead to the outputs?
- What combination of learning methods?

Planning the venue

- Is access adequate (e.g. travel and stairs)?
- Residential?
- What atmosphere is required? Seating arrangements? Flip-charts? Tables?
- Facilities – Refreshments? Toilets? Equipment? Materials? Syndicate rooms?

Information

- Explanatory literature – what the event is, why it is important, directions.
- Personal recruitment of those you particularly want to attend.
- Conference pack and draft post-conference follow-up information.

Plan follow-through

- Rehearse at the outset various options for carrying forwards the outputs from the meeting.
- How to keep the database of participants updated?
- What expectations about ongoing relationships?

Visualisation

- Talk through the programme minute by minute with your team.
- Physically walk through the venue and sit in the chairs – what does it feel like?
- Talk through intended follow-up with your team – can you deliver what you promise?

Centring the learning space: the story, energisers, ground rules, evaluation

Participants need to locate themselves in a shared story – to be 'on the same page'. They need to agree where they are in this story. They need to: be ready to engage; know what to expect from others; and be confident that it is valuable. This scene-setting activity can take a few minutes, and it can take hours or days. If it is overly rushed you lose time overall, because misunderstandings slow things at a later stage. If it is overly slow people become bored and distracted. Leaders make judgements about what is optimal, and adjust in-the-moment if their original expectation turns out to be wrong.

Agreeing the stage of the story

Participants need a succinct summary of what is known and unknown about the past and future, and what the meeting is expected to contribute to both. They need to know when the meeting will end and what will happen afterwards. Leaders at meetings gain agreement from participants about this analysis before continuing. This entails:

- written literature to read beforehand
- checking with the whole group at the start of the meeting
- acknowledgement from the front who is present, and who is not.

Energisers

In the same way that athletes warm up their body, participants need to warm up their minds to be ready for creative interaction. This means that they need to be physically comfortable (a cold room can greatly slow things down) and to 'hear their voice in the room'. They also need to interact with each other, finding and creating rapport at an early stage, and also later on. An energiser can help all of these at the same time. It entails:

- introducing each other – possibly in small groups
- a game appropriate to the meeting (introductions in small group can be enough).

Ground rules

Participants need to know what is acceptable behaviour. It can be helpful to give a general statement about meeting behaviour at the beginning of a meeting (e.g. mobile phones). Immediately before attempting exercises that might make people feel vulnerable a deeper exploration and agreement. For example, before under-taking role-play, the leader of a meeting must make sure that the group as a whole agrees the ground rules. This entails:

- a statement that ground rules are needed as a safety net
- participants generate or revisit ground rules before 'risky' exercises such as role play.

Evaluation

To 'evaluate' means to find the value of something. Different people value different things. The participants must learn things of use to them. The funders need to see that the purpose has been achieved. You need insights into how you are fulfilling your role. Meetings are a good opportunity to agree all these domains of evaluation, to gain instant data about them, and also to gain agreement about what later data participants will provide. This entails:

- clarifying to all what different things need to be evaluated for what purpose
- retaining evaluation data – flip-chart notes, evaluation sheets, plenary agreements.

Small-group–large-group iterations

Small-group–large-group iterations create ownership and energy. In small groups participants generate a breadth of ideas. To avoid boredom feedback should include only a few ideas sufficient to move towards whole-group consensus.

The breadth of participant ideas can be gathered from a wall of comments, as used in 'Future search', through group summary sheets as used in 'Open space' and through flip-chart recording.

Here, I describe the use of prepared questions for small-group discussion with flip-chart recording. The flip charts are later written up and attached as an appendix to the conference report. This is distributed soon after the event to retain momentum and clarify disagreements. A planning group moves things forwards before the next meeting.

Helping participants to engage in small groups quickly

- Participants will enthusiastically engage when they see the value of an exercise, when they can easily understand what is asked of them, and when there is an empowering atmosphere. Explaining clearly how the small group work contributes to the whole conference, easy-to-understand directions and good facilitation help these.
- You give instructions verbally in plenary session and also in writing (e.g. on paper, flip charts or a wall). Depending on the situation you may want to agree beforehand group facilitators and rapporteurs; alternatively, you can ask each group to appoint their own.
- Each group needs their own flip chart and different coloured pens that *work*. They must know that 'if it gets written down it gets written up'. Contributions should be written as intelligible sentences.
- One group member is invited to give a brief plenary insight into their conversation to get a flavour of the group conclusions. Asking them to feedback only one idea from the last question can often do this.

A sequence of ideas

- It often helps for a conference to start with an exercise in developing shared vision, before focusing on detailed practicalities. This helps to avoid the (often huge) practical obstacles to success from obstructing imaginative thinking. For example, the first session might agree what world participants want to create, the second session identifies obstacles to achieving this, and the third develops a plan for practical next steps.

- In each session three sequential questions help to build from individual experience to conference recommendations. The first question invites participants to give a personal anecdote relevant to the situation and the third invites recommendations for action. The second links the other two.

Examples of a question sequence

- When gaining expectation at the start of a conference it might be: Who am I?', 'What is my interest in this topic?' and 'What do I want from the conference?'
- When prioritising goals it might be: 'What goals do I think are important?', 'Which of these are feasible within resources?' and 'What goals do we recommend?'
- When exploring how to achieve a conference goal it might be: 'Obstacles to success?', 'Potential solutions to these obstacles?' and 'Recommendations for conference?'
- When building from the ideas suggested in other groups it might be: 'In what ways are our ideas relevant to the ideas of other groups?', 'What changes to our ideas do we wish to make?' and 'What further negotiations do we need to find a win–win?'

Chapter 17

Seeing things through different eyes

Summary

Integrated primary health care must incorporate multiple different perspectives. We are all trapped inside our own ways of seeing the world. These come from our ideas, histories, skills and ambitions. Leadership challenges practitioners and managers to work for the system as a whole. This does not mean that we have to put aside our preferred ways of seeing things, but it does mean that we have to value what others see. For this we each need some insight into what it is like to 'see' through different eyes, and feel through different skin.

In this chapter I describe four techniques that help to do this. They are:

- Personal visualisation – rehearsing in your mind what you will do in real life.
- Vision workshop – groups of people go on an imaginary journey into the future and later describe the insights they gain.
- Role-play and scenarios – a facilitator sets a scene in which people adopt unfamiliar roles. They rehearse the scene, or a sequence of scenes, then de-role and discuss what insights they gained.
- Fish bowl – a small number of people in a circle discuss something of importance, surrounded by observers. Rules govern entering and exiting the bowl.

Personal visualisation

What this is trying to achieve

Visualisation helps your subconscious mental models to prepare yourself to succeed in something you have to do. It could be a job interview, a talk or a meeting.

Visualisation is more than a rehearsal of the words you will say. It is a subconscious role-play of the whole situation. It includes how you will feel about yourself, the impression you want others to gain and the outcomes you expect. Before you start you need an idea of what you want to achieve. Many visualisations have been described for use in everyday life (see *Stepping Into the Magic – A New Approach to Everyday Life*).[1]

Instructions

- Find a quiet place where you will not be disturbed and make yourself comfortable. You may like to sit in a chair or lie on the floor. Perhaps take your shoes off, or wear a blindfold. If you want you can set an alarm for 30 minutes.
- First, quickly imagine in as much detail as you can what it is you hope to achieve. Then put this out of your mind (don't worry, it will come back later, and in a more coherent form).
- Close your eyes and stretch then relax the muscles of your whole body. Start at the head and neck, then shoulders and arms . . . Continue down your body to your toes. If muscles become tense again, focus on these, and if necessary repeat the whole body exercise.
- Listen to the furthermost sounds you can hear. Spend some time mentally outside of the room listening to them. Then put them out of your mind.
- Listen to the noises close to you. Be conscious of your breathing. Then put these also out of your mind.
- Then talk yourself into a subconscious journey. First imagine yourself descending in some way. You may prefer to feel yourself falling, or going down an escalator, or a lift. Feel an altered state of consciousness come over you.
- Alternatively you may find it helpful to repeat the word re-lax several times, then slowly count yourself down from ten to one.
- You arrive in a peaceful place. In this place you feel confident and fully yourself. It may have visual features – a garden, seaside, mountain. If these come allow them, but if they don't it does not matter. You are ready to start the visualisation.
- Search your mind's eye for the situation you are concerned about. When you find it ask your subconscious to give you an image of it. If no image comes let yourself *feel* it in some other way. Look at the surroundings – the rooms, the furniture, the people.
- When ready, let the scenario unfold. First, feel your way into each person in the room. What is their interest in this? What other related concerns do they have? What approach from you will appeal to them?
- Then focus on yourself. Engage with each of the individuals and the whole group. Remove from what you intended to say the things that will turn them away. Be reasonable, balanced, and invincible. Use humour, anger and calm argument appropriate to the context. Watch yourself achieve the things you want. Watch them agree. Note where they do not.
- When you are finished listen to what each of them has to say to you. When neither you nor they have anything else to say, say goodbye, thanking your subconscious for the experience.
- Allow yourself to come back to the room. One way is to count from one to five, suggesting to yourself that when you reach five you will be wide awake, refreshed and at peace.
- You may find it helpful to write notes about what you have learnt. When doing it for real remember to use the things you have learnt.

Vision workshop

What this is trying to achieve

A vision workshop helps a group of people to go on an imaginary journey into the future to see what integrated primary health care would look like. The following is a model we often used in Liverpool.[2] As Weisbord and Janoff point out, asking participants to visualise the future can result in two unhelpful polarities – an overly pessimistic extension of the problems perceived at the time, or a utopian extreme where there are no problems.[3] You can help to overcome these two extremes by using the 'appreciative enquiry' technique of building future vision from existing things that work (Chapter 15). Participants put themselves five, ten or 20 years into the future 'as if they have made their dreams come true'.

This exercise is a subconscious role-play of the evolving story that helps participants to decide next steps that are coherent with past success and future hopes.

Instructions

- Find a large comfortable room (not too much echo or disturbance). Invite participants to make themselves comfortable, perhaps on chairs or lying on the floor. You are the journey facilitator. Use a calm, soft and measured voice throughout.
- Invite participants to close their eyes, take a few deep breaths and then stretch the muscles of the whole body. Start at the head and neck, then shoulders and arms . . . continue to the toes, relaxing the muscles after tensing them. Slow down or speed up your narrative as you think necessary.
- Invite participant to listen to the furthermost sounds, out of the room, and then put them out of their minds.
- Invite participants to listen to the closest sounds – then put them out of their minds.
- Invite participants to be conscious of their breathing – calm, peaceful and safe.
- Tell them they are going down in an escalator. Down and down and down . . . perfectly safe.
- You tell them that they arrive in a peaceful place where they feel confident and fully alive. It may have visual features – a garden, seaside, a mountain. It may not. It does not matter. They are ready to start the visualisation.
- Invite participants to arrive in the situation they want to explore, perhaps their town in ten years' time. Tell them that all their dreams for integrated primary health care have come true. They can arrive any way they like – on foot, by air or any other way. Ask them what they see and what it feels like. Invite them to travel around the town to see other things. Ask them to observe other things, both good and bad, that are consequences of their success. Leave participants in their imaginations for a while – perhaps five minutes – until it seems to you that they have seen enough.
- When it seems time, invite participants to come back to the room in their own time, arriving wide awake and refreshed.
- When everyone is back, invite immediate comments from all parts of the room. Give them the option to write down what they saw before they forget. Then discuss in groups.

Role-play, scenarios and simulations

What this is trying to achieve

Role-plays, scenarios and simulations help participants to experience a complex, threatening or risky situation in relative safety. This does not mean that it is completely safe and you must make sure that good ground rules are agreed, and you have access to extricate people from potentially damaging situations. They are helpful to rehearse real-life situations, such as job interviews or presentations.

I have found them very helpful to improve funding proposals (e.g. for research and audit projects). First, I get the whole group to agree criteria for a good proposal, and then split them into applicants and an interview panel. Each applicant (or team) presents their proposal and the panel question them according to the criteria. After the applicants have presented their proposals I facilitate a goldfish bowl where the panel discusses the merits of each proposal. Then the roles are reversed. Finally, they discuss in one large group what they have learnt.

A scenario is more complicated than a simple role play because different groups have different tasks and after an initial scene, they go away to amend their plans in the light of the first discussion, coming back to role-play another scene. This works well when devising a complex intervention or negotiating a way forward with multiple constituencies. It helps to give one group the role to help the other groups with their plans and to spring surprises on them, by changing the rules of engagement at short notice. A simulation is a real-life scenario.

Instructions for a scenario

- Explain to the whole group the issues to be discussed. Let us take the example of evaluating the impact of an intervention. Different groups (perhaps three) are asked to devise proposals using different research approaches, or to represent different constituencies. Another group is the funding panel and a fifth is a design group.
- Give each group time to develop their plans (say, 20 minutes). The first three groups present in turn their ideas to the panel who question them. The other groups watch. If time permits the panel can discuss the applications among themselves in a goldfish bowl, watched by all the groups.
- The design group then tells the whole room (or the panel if you prefer) new information that alters the goals (e.g. more or less money, a new policy directive or a crisis). The panel debates and then gives new instructions to the three groups to rewrite their proposals.
- A further period of planning takes place before the next presentations.
- A variation of this could allow interaction between the three groups of applicants to draw on each others' strengths.
- At the end the facilitator invites each group in turn what they have learnt before opening the discussion out to the whole room.

Common mistakes

- Giving imprecise instructions.
- Using a role play/scenario that is overly confronting for the group.
- Forgetting to de-role.

Fish bowl

What this is trying to achieve

A fish bowl prompts group members to take responsibility for their thoughts and actions. It helps them to listen well to others, and also to listen better to what they themselves are saying. It makes them better aware that they impact on others, and that others are really treating them seriously. It does this by holding conversations in public that are usually held in private.

This is useful in training courses and teambuilding workshops, both as a role-play to rehearse difficult situations, and to agree ground rules between people who will have to work together. It can also be used in real-life situations such as to observe a senior management team discussing strategic issues in front of other team members. The Merseyside GP Registrar Course Organisers devised a powerful variation that involved goldfish bowls inside goldfish bowls inside goldfish bowls – so everyone was both observed and observer.

Instructions

- Arrange seats in a circle according to the number of people to enter the goldfish bowl, plus one or two extra seats.
- Arrange seats or standing spaces in places of your choosing around the bowl for the observers.
- Explain to the whole group the issue to be discussed. The issue should come from the group. If a 'real' situation the outcomes of the group discussions must be consequential, and final decisions must not already have been made. For example, it could be priorities for development, allocation of funds, or solving complex problems. The group must agree ground rules, understanding that they are seeing only a snapshot of the issue that must not later be taken out of context. The observers are not allowed to talk or otherwise distract those inside the goldfish bowl.
- You invite the discussants to enter the goldfish bowl and to start their conversation. Agree someone to step into your role of facilitating the session if you have to enter the bowl for any reason.
- Agree with the discussants rules about the use of the spare seat(s). One of the seats is for you, in case you feel a need to join them to deal with a problem or to stimulate them in another direction. If observers are allowed to enter the goldfish bowl to contribute, the conditions under which they can do this, and how long they can stay, must be agreed.
- Allow the conversation to start. At the appropriate time enter the bowl yourself to call time on the exercise.
- A modification of the exercise allows the observers to act as consultants. Behind each discussant is an observer/consultant. At agreed times the internal participants can consult with this person. 'Consultants' are not allowed to enter into the discussion, only advising their partner to contribute effectively. These roles can be reversed later.
- At the end first ask the discussants to 'shake off' the role and ask for their reflections. Second, and only after *all* discussants have had a chance to speak, invite observers to contribute to the discussions about learning gained from the exercise.

Common mistakes

- Inadequate understanding of the rules results in loss of flow.
- Getting stranded from a problem.
- Allowing the observers to speak before the discussants.

References

1 Edwards G (1996) *Stepping Into the Magic – A New Approach to Everyday Life*. Piatkus, London.
2 Sainsbury P and Dowrick C (1995) Vision workshops – a planning tool for general practice. *Education in General Practice*. **6**: 62–8.
3 Weisbord M and Janoff S (2000) *Future Search – An Action Guide to Finding Common Ground in Organizations and Communities*. Berrett-Koehler, San Francisco, CA.

Chapter 18

Interviewing for team players

Summary

The chapter describes two techniques to assess how candidates will perform as team players by role-playing real life situations.

Getting the right person first time pays back the effort you put in many times over. There are many aspects of good interviewing techniques that are targeted at individual assessment. These include comparing the skills of the candidate with the job description and person specifications, and social/psychological/learning profiles of Belbin, Myers Briggs, and Honey and Mumford.

In this chapter I describe two techniques I have used many times with good effect. They put candidates into a group situation where they encounter the kind of situations they might encounter in real life. They are:

- Assessing shared leadership skills – using a combination of small group interaction, formal presentation and reflection on performance to gain multiple insights into the flexibility and breadth of someone's skills.
- In-tray tests – observing candidates (especially administration staff) doing the tasks they will do in the real job.

These techniques help you to better see what people actually do in situations, rather than what they say they do. It helps not only to get the 'best candidate' but also the best make-up of teams. They are useful both to test how someone will fit into an existing team, and also how new teams can be employed at the same time.

Both techniques involve asking each candidate at formal interview (usually on the following day for shared leadership skills) about their performance. This reveals their skills of self-reflection. It also commonly offers insight into why they performed the way they did (good or bad) on the previous day. Both successful and unsuccessful candidates usually report satisfaction with the process because the process is so transparent.

Assessing shared leadership skills

What this is trying to achieve

This is a technique that helps to identify people with the potential to be members of leadership teams. It looks not for one personality type, but for the skills of adapting to new people and contexts, able to listen, appreciate and reflect. It can also reveal what combination of people will work well together in a team. It gains multiple insights into people through observing their performance in small groups, rehearsed presentation and formal interview. This combination of insight helps the appointing group to see something of the flexibility and breadth of their skills. I have successfully used this model for the simultaneous appointment of 20 people for four teams, as well as for single posts. Almost always with hindsight we felt we made the right choices. Almost always even the candidates who failed to get the posts felt that they were given a fair chance to display themselves (one even volunteered that she 'went home singing').

Instructions

- Decide the job description and personal specifications in the usual way.
- Explain in writing that the interview will take place on two days and involve three stages. The first day will take up to four hours and in this part they will be in the company of the other candidates. It will involve group work and a presentation. On the second day they will have a formal interview that will take about 20 minutes, when they will be alone with the panel. For the second part of the first day ask candidates to prepare a presentation of five minutes on something they did that they are proud of, and that shows why they would be good for the post. Hire a large room or hall for the first day.
- On the first day you will need two facilitator/interviewers per eight candidates, plus one extra who holds it all together. In a large circle first invite everyone to introduce themselves and to ask questions about the post. Continue until all questions are finished.
- Invite the candidates to join pre-decided groups of eight around a flip chart (separated far enough apart to prevent interference). If there is an odd number, or fewer than four people, ask your team members to make up the numbers; if they are more than eight candidates split the groups. Each circle has one of your facilitators/interviewers inside the circle and another outside. Both have a list of things to score the candidates that come from the personal specifications. I usually use a different template for the internal and external interviewers to get different kinds of snapshots of the individuals.
- The internal facilitator asks the participants to form pairs. Each has two minutes to explain to their partner a success story, then change roles. A big clock on the wall helps. When finished (five minutes) candidates take it in turn to tell the story of their partner to the whole group. Then the group as a whole debates the general lessons from the stories as a whole. The internal facilitator/ interviewer gives little guidance about how to do this and waits to see what happens – he or she can be more directive if they get stuck. It takes about 45 minutes. Both facilitator/interviewers make notes and scores about each candidate.
- They break for tea. Then each candidate presents their work using audio-visual aids of their choice (I am always surprised at how different these can be and how clever people are at choosing methods that suit them). Again they are scored for this.
- After the candidates have gone, the facilitator/interviewers meet together and discuss each candidate in turn. Scores are compared and charted.
- At formal interview the next day, one or two of the previous day's facilitator/ interviewers are present, and there are new interviewers on the panel. The

scores are considered and areas to explore further are identified before each candidate enters. The first question is how they think they did on the previous day (this often immediately addresses the things the panel wanted to explore). It reveals their ability to reflect and learn as well as whether they really want the job. The panel takes the final decision, mindful of the balance of evidence.

In-tray tests

What this is trying to achieve

In-tray tests are an attempt to put candidates into the situation they are likely to be in, if they were to be appointed. This is particularly useful for administration roles. By involving your team members in designing the tests and evaluating the candidates you are also using it as a team-building exercise. This also signals to candidates and your team the culture that you wish to develop. As well as evaluating task skills, this approach can reveal team skills and which candidates will best fit with your team.

Instructions

- Write the job description and personal specifications in the usual way.
- Involve your team in the development of the in-tray tests. They include about five tasks, such as searching for information from a set of books, typing from a tape, typesetting a document, making a telephone call, filing. Write the list down. Ask candidates to have a go at all of them, and not to spend too long on any one.
- Use a team member to welcome the candidate and chat with the intention of reducing nerves.
- When ready, the candidate goes to the 'interview' room where the tasks are explained by the most senior facilitator/interviewer, who then leaves them to do this. Another team member remains in the room to help with any difficulties.
- The candidate undertakes the tasks observed by a second team member who also continues with their own work.
- At the appropriate time (say, 15 minutes) the senior person comes back in and asks how it went. The 'answers' to the in-tray tests are gathered and looked at.
- Your whole team convenes and each candidate is considered, comparing the objective and subjective evidence from different teams members about their performance.
- The candidates have formal interviews (possibly later that day).

A final word

When I was eight years old my father died, aged 37. He was a GP who worked alone in Merthyr Tydfil, South Wales – one of the most deprived towns in the UK. It happened on 4 April 1963, when the thaw came after a most severe winter. Three weeks earlier a fellow GP had also died. Five days after my father's death another GP dropped dead, as it happened on his way to my father's funeral. Throughout those frozen months they had done house calls on foot since the roads were impassable, often walking late at night in the mountains with medical bags in hand. All these good men were from the small Borough of Merthyr alone.

The diagnosis of heart attack on each of their death certificates did no justice to the complexity of the causes. Twenty children were orphaned. In those days in Merthyr there was no primary care organisation to plan manpower, or locum agency to provide backup. None of the families even thought it wrong at the time – complete commitment to patients came with the job, whatever the personal cost.

In my child's mind I promised myself that I would under no circumstances ever become a doctor, and especially not a GP. It was only the unattractiveness of other university options that made me a reluctant medical student. A completely unplanned and unexpected series of coincidences led me to later take the path I did.

Yet only recently did I make the connection between my childhood loss and the fact that I have devoted most of my adult life to making general practice better.

Funny thing, hidden motivations.

Index